# IMPORTANT ORAL AND MAXILLOFACIAL PRESENTATIONS
## for the Primary Care Clinician

Alexander M C Goodson

Arpan S Tahim

Karl F B Payne

Peter A Brennan

Published in 2016 by Libri Publishing

ISBN 978-1-909818-93-4

Cover and Design by Carnegie Book Production


Printed in the UK by Hobbs the Printers

Libri Publishing
Brunel House
Volunteer Way
Faringdon
Oxfordshire
SN7 7YR

Tel: +44 (0)845 873 3837

www.libripublishing.co.uk

**Acknowledgements**
*The authors wish to thank all patients involved for permitting the use of clinical
photographs in this book. Thanks also to Peter Sims, the GP representative,
BAOMS and the RCGP for supporting this initiative. Finally, thanks also to the
authors' partners (Claire, Susan, Caroline and Rachel) and families for their
ongoing support.*

## FOREWORD

Oral and maxillofacial conditions presenting in General Practice can be challenging to identify and manage. This book provides readily accessible information that reinforces learning through different ways.

The many photographs in the book supports the 'Ask, Look and Do' approach that the authors advocate when faced with such clinical conditions. The importance of a good clinical examination is a common thread throughout the book.

The range of conditions that we are faced with in General Practice is wide and the book presents these in logical themed chapters. A particular feature is recognition of conditions that warrant immediate referral or referral through cancer pathways supported by a traffic light approach and the algorithms which provide an easily readable and logical approach to decision making.

What is good to see is that there is some discussion on atypical presentations (e.g. facial pain) which we know can be challenging to treat and manage.

This book will have longevity and will be invaluable to medical students, those in training or in established practice.

I congratulate Professor Peter Brennan and his team on producing this thoughtful and practical resource.

Dr Imran Rafi BSc MBBS MRCGP FRCP MSc PhD

**GP Principal and Chair of the RCGP
Clinical Innovation and Research Centre**

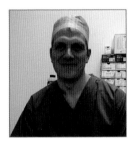

**Mr Alexander M C Goodson BSc(Hons) MBBS BDS MRCS DOHNS**

Specialty Trainee in Oral and Maxillofacial Surgery, Wales Deanery

**Mr Arpan S Tahim BSc(Hons) MBBS BDS MRCS MEd**

Specialty Trainee in Oral and Maxillofacial Surgery, London Deanery

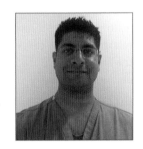

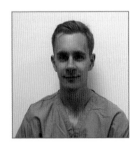

**Mr Karl F B Payne BMedSci(Hons) BMBS BDS MRCS**

Specialty Trainee in Oral and Maxillofacial Surgery, West Midlands Deanery

**Prof Peter A Brennan MD FRCS FRCSI FDS**

Consultant Oral and Maxillofacial Surgeon, President British Association of Oral and Maxillofacial Surgeons

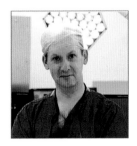

# CONTENTS

# PREFACE

I am delighted to have been asked to provide the preface for *Important Oral and Maxillofacial Presentations for the Primary Care Clinician*. The British Association of Oral and Maxillofacial Surgeons (BAOMS) is proud to fund this book as part Professor Peter Brennan's BAOMS Presidential programme. Peter has thought beyond his immediate colleagues' needs and developed a source that helps inform patient management at a primary care level. By using his presidential fund for the development and publication of this book, he and his co-authors (who are trainees in our specialty) will help the busy generalist diagnose and manage oro-facial conditions (including the less common malignancies). With his unique collaboration with the Royal College of General Practitioners and distributing the material free to practitioners and trainees, Peter is providing a legacy that will improve patient care long after his term of office is finished.

As one expects of a journal editor, the text is clearly and logically set out supported by relevant illustrations; the result is a very accessible resource. The book is an example of an excellent collaboration between primary and secondary care clinicians to assist in improving patient care. I know Peter is the first to acknowledge the hard work put in by his team of Alexander Goodson, Arpan Tahim and Karl Payne.

The various chapters enable clinicians to diagnose oro-facial conditions and, where needed, accelerate appropriate referrals. The use of colour-coded, highlighted bullet points for urgent referrals e.g. possible head and neck cancers, helps clinicians in a very practical way. The text is clear and the use of algorithms both in the book and accompanying poster directs the busy practitioner.

Using the book in combination with support from local specialist Oral and Maxillofacial Surgeons will undoubtedly assist you in ensuring a speedy effective care pathway for your patients. I unhesitatingly recommend this book and would suggest you share with as many of your colleagues and trainees as possible.

**Mike Davidson FDS RCS (Lond.) FRCS (Edin.)**

**Chairman of the Council British Association of Oral and Maxillofacial Surgeons. London**

# INTRODUCTION

Head and neck cancer is an important and serious condition. Its incidence is increasing year by year in the UK. Given its anatomical location with so many important structures in such a confined area, treatment options (and surgery in particular) can have a significant risk of morbidity and mortality, with potentially disastrous psychosocial consequences to patients, their relatives and friends. It commonly presents late or in advanced stages, making it difficult to treat, leading to a poorer prognosis.

Understanding the head, neck and oral cavity can be daunting for the Primary Care Clinician. These anatomical regions of the body seem to lack the same emphasis during medical undergraduate and postgraduate training, and the oral cavity in particular can be extremely unfamiliar for many general medical practitioners. For dentists, head and neck anatomy teaching is often focused on the lower third of the facial skeleton and dental tissues, with less emphasis on other anatomical regions and soft tissue anatomy.

This book aims to simplify the face, mouth and neck for the Primary Care Clinician by providing a brief, presentation-based account of important oral and maxillofacial conditions that are likely to be encountered in primary care. Furthermore, we have tried to highlight those presentations that are dangerous and should prompt rapid onward referral through a cancer referral pathway to secondary care.

Each chapter begins with a brief introduction, followed by an ASK → LOOK → DO structure to guide the clinician to an appropriate management/referral option. We summarise key questions to ASK during the history-taking process and important features to LOOK for during an examination. For each presentation, we outline important SINISTER FEATURES that should make you suspicious of potentially malignant disease. This is followed by a simple, easy-to-follow 'DO' management algorithm in a standard format throughout which aims to consolidate the relevant information gained during the history and examination. These algorithms should provide you with one of several management options including

- Urgent cancer referral
- Routine referral

- Immediate referral to on-call oral and maxillofacial (OMFS) team
- Referral to local dental practitioner
- Management in primary care (i.e. General Medical Practitioner, General Dental Practitioner or other Primary Care Clinician as appropriate).

Each chapter then explains these diagnoses and management processes in greater detail.

This book (with accompanying algorithms) is by no means exhaustive and does not include all the pathology encountered in this region. Neither will it provide an in-depth or detailed understanding of the oral cavity and its dental aspects. However, by exploring the various important OMFS presentations in this way, we hope to provide you with a useful, practical outline with a focus on detection of potentially malignant disease, while providing a framework for management for other relevant conditions.

# CHAPTER 1:
# EXAMINATION

As with all conditions, the cornerstone of management of oral and facial pathology, and in particular the safe management of potential malignancy, lies in taking a good history and performing a thorough examination.

Although the oral cavity and face (and to a lesser extent the neck) are unfamiliar to many healthcare professionals, the principles of history taking are similar to those most of us are familiar with and will not be covered further.

The same cannot be said for the examination of the oral cavity and face, which is the focus of this chapter. A simple examination of the dental hard tissues, the oral soft tissues, face and neck will be outlined below.

## INTRA-ORAL EXAMINATION

An adult with a full dentition will have 32 teeth. These are divided into four quadrants, each containing from the midline outwards: a central incisor, lateral incisor, a canine, 2 premolar teeth and 3 molar teeth (Fig 1.1). The last of these molar teeth are often called wisdom teeth, and can be absent. Aside from dental pathology, many soft tissue pathologies can be described in relation to the dentition so it is useful to be able to accurately describe it.

While a detailed dental examination is routine in primary dental care, it is not feasible in a general medical practice setting. Therefore, a sensible brief examination would include:

a) observation of significant dental decay/discolouration and the presence of plastic, ceramic or metal fillings and crowns
b) palpation to elicit increased mobility of teeth
c) percussion for tenderness (tapping the upper surface of a tooth)
d) looking to see if there are any discharging gum boils (sinuses) on the gums which are a sign of chronic dental root (apical) infection.

The manner in which the patient's teeth meet/bite together (dental occlusion) can also give useful information about the underlying pathology. Although beyond the scope of this book, in the primary care setting,

EXAMINATION

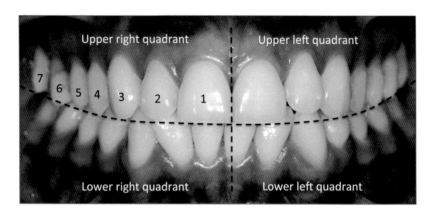

*Fig 1.1: Labelling the quadrants of the mouth and numbering the teeth*

1. *Central incisor*
2. *Lateral incisor*
3. *Canine*
4. *First premolar*
5. *Second premolar*
6. *First molar*
7. *Second molar*
8. *Third molar/ wisdom tooth (missing in this patient)*

it should be noted if the patient feels that their occlusion (or 'bite') has changed.

In addition, a thorough intra-oral examination requires systematic assessment of all mucosal surfaces (Fig 1.2). These areas include:

- buccal mucosa (inner lining of cheek), including the opening of parotid duct opposite the upper second molar
- labial mucosa (inner surface of lips)
- gingival surfaces (gums) – including looking for gum boils (sinuses) mentioned above
- hard palate
- soft palate
- tongue (dorsal surface, lateral border and ventral aspect)
- floor of mouth
- oropharynx
- retromolar region (area of mucosa just behind the last standing molar tooth).

a

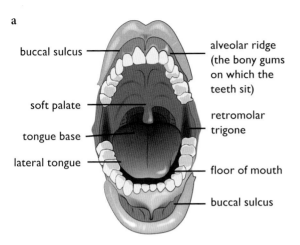

buccal sulcus

alveolar ridge
(the bony gums
on which the
teeth sit)

soft palate

retromolar
trigone

tongue base

lateral tongue

floor of mouth

buccal sulcus

EXAMINATION

*Fig 1.2a: Key anatomical sites to examine in the oral cavity.*

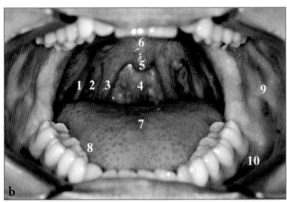

b

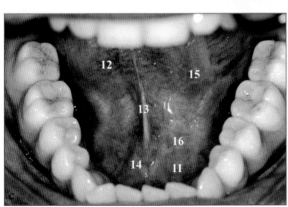

c

*Fig 1.2: b) Intraoral and c) floor of mouth anatomy. The parotid duct (Stenson's duct) drains via the parotid papilla, which is out of sight, opposite the upper second molar teeth bilaterally:*

1. Palatoglossal arch
2. Palatine tonsil
3. Palatopharyngeal arch
4. Posterior pharyngeal wall
5. Uvula
6. Soft palate
7. Dorsum of tongue
8. Lateral border of tongue
9. Buccal mucosa
10. Buccal sulcus
11. Floor of mouth
12. Ventral surface of tongue
13. Lingual fraenum
14. Submandibular duct openings
15. Lingual vein
16. Sublingual fold

EXAMINATION

Although the confined nature of the oral cavity, along with the various 'obstacles' such as the tongue and teeth, can make it difficult to visualise certain areas, they can generally be examined without any specialist equipment other than good lighting and a wooden tongue spatula. At this stage, it would be prudent to assess for lower lip and tongue numbness along with tongue protrusion.

As with any examination, any lesion found in the mouth should be observed and palpated to establish their site, size, shape, colour and nature of their borders, along with associated regional lymphadenopathy and assessment for any neurological sequelae.

## FACIAL AND NECK EXAMINATION

A basic facial examination includes observation at rest, assessing for objective facial asymmetry arising from, for example facial swellings, muscle hypertrophy or one-sided facial weakness. Close observation of the jaw can give important insight into the temporomandibular joint (TMJ). The extent of mouth opening can be noted, along with any jaw deviation. Assessment of jaw protrusion and lateral movements can give further information about the function of the TMJ. Facial weakness can be assessed at this stage in the standard manner.

Underlying bony prominences and skeletal deformity should be palpated and asymmetry noted. Important areas include the nasal bones, malar prominences, supraorbital rims, the lateral orbital rim, infraorbital rim, zygomatic arch prominences and the mandible. Crepitus (similar to any other superficial joint) from the TMJ on opening/closing the jaw can be noted. The masseter and temporalis muscles are palpated for tenderness passively, during jaw movements and on clenching. The lateral pterygoid muscles can be felt intra-orally by pressing posteriorly in the upper buccal sulcus. The medial pterygoid muscle can be palpated for tenderness just underneath (medial to) the angle of the mandible. Soft tissue lumps and lesions on the face should follow the same examination protocol – assessment of site, size, shape, colour, consistency, nature of their borders, regional lymphadenopathy and any associated neurology. The site of suspected lymphadenopathy is best described according to its anatomical level (Ia, Ib, IIa, IIb, etc.). These levels are illustrated in Figure 1.3

The nose should be assessed for deformity and patency to breathing (closing each nostril separately and asking the patient to breathe through the other). Intra-nasal examination can easily be performed with an otoscope (preferably with the aid of a nasal speculum if available), looking for any intranasal deformity, swellings, ulceration or signs of recent bleeding.

The principles of a good neck examination will be familiar to you and the standard inspection and palpation sequence should be followed. Observation might highlight any areas of concern and examination of lumps and lesions can be described in terms of their site, size, shape, colour, consistency, nature of their borders, trans-illuminesence (though rarely used in the head and neck) and assessed in relation to swallowing and tongue protrusion. As many doctors, dentists and allied professionals are comfortable examining the neck, the fine details will not be covered further in this book. However, it should be stressed that if a neck examination reveals lymphadenopathy, it is imperative to examine the oral cavity, nose and face for potential sources of malignancy, and where appropriate, the other lymph node sites (axilla, groin) and abdomen as well for generalised lymphadenopathy or organomegaly.

This basic examination sequence is not exhaustive and the examination should be tailored to each patient's presenting features. Further eye, ear or cranial nerve assessment may be indicated at the practitioner's discretion. However, this simple framework will hopefully be useful to you in the following chapters, as the important presentations in the orofacial region are explored in greater detail.

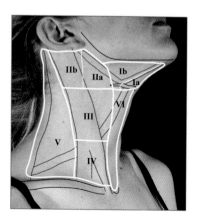

*Fig 1.3: Lymph node levels of the neck, with basic representation of underlying anatomy. The widely used levels of the neck are also marked.*

# CHAPTER 2:
# ORAL ULCERS

ORAL ULCERS

## INTRODUCTION

An ulcer is a break in the continuity of the epithelial surface due to progressive tissue destruction. Morphology of oral ulcers can be hugely variable, as can the underlying aetiology. It is therefore important to not only clinically examine the ulcer's appearance and site, but also the history of its behaviour. Relapsing-remitting or recurrent ulcers often have different aetiology to persistent ulcers, or those appearing in a single episode, as do solitary ulcers compared to those appearing in crops.

The presence of particular sinister features (including risk factors) will direct towards urgent management. Their absence however will enable the Primary Care Clinician to take a rational, safe and stepwise approach to investigation and management.

This chapter looks to identify key points to assess in the history and important features on examination. This management algorithm uses **pain** as its keystone and then defines an ulcer as **persistent**, **recurrent** or **solitary**. By using this logical approach in primary care, you will arrive at the correct referral outcome.

**ASK:**
- Risk factor assessment
- Painful vs. painless
- Duration (< / > 3 weeks?)
- Persistent vs. recurrent
- Solitary or multiple
- Previous history of oral cancer
- Medications – nicorandil/aspirin
- Associated with other systemic symptoms – ulcers in other areas (e.g. skin, genital, corneal)
- PMH of autoimmune disease

## LOOK:

- Size (less than or greater than 10mm)
- Site (high risk areas for malignancy: tongue, retromolar, attached gingiva [non-mobile gum])
- Features – shape, colour, edge, surrounding induration, base/depth of invasion
- Obvious traumatic cause (e.g. teeth/fillings with sharp edges?)
- Nearby teeth deviated? Loose?
- Palpate for lymphadenopathy

## SINISTER FEATURES:

- Extending beyond mucosa
- Irregular border
- Firm/indurated
- Associated neck lymphadenopathy – single or more than one node
- Nerve weakness/altered sensation
- Not healed after >3 weeks
- On high-risk areas (lateral tongue, floor of mouth, anterior and base of tongue, retromolar, tonsils, oropharynx [back of throat], attached gingiva, palate, floor of mouth and lip)
- Painless ulcer
- Loose/missing/deviated teeth
- Previous oral cancer history
- Risk factor history (smoking, alcohol, betel nut chewing)

ORAL ULCERS

# DO: MANAGEMENT ALGORITHM

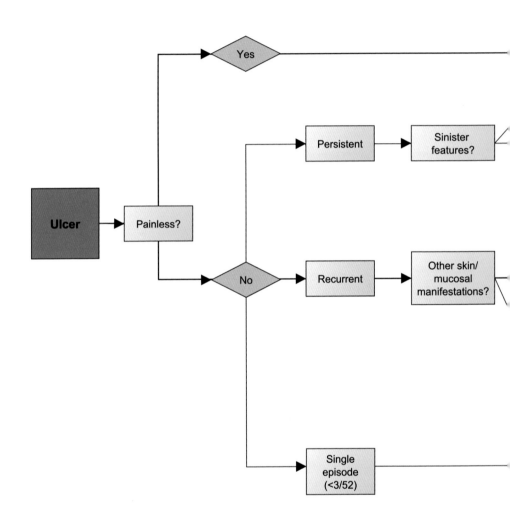

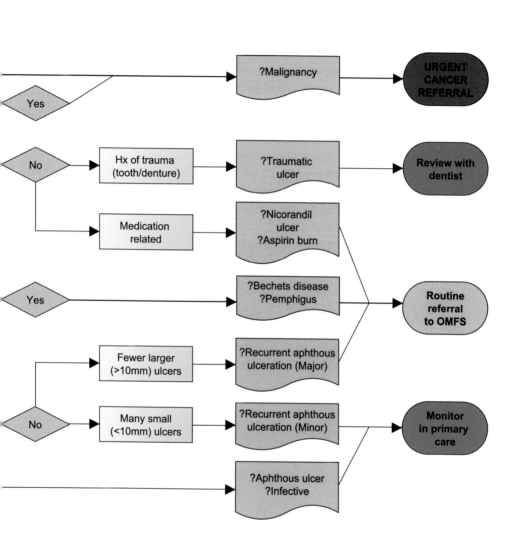

## URGENT CANCER REFERRAL

### SUSPICIOUS ULCERS

Up to 95% of oral cancers are squamous cell carcinomas (SCC). These cancers typically present as a persistent, destructive yet relatively painless, firm and indurated mouth ulcer (present for more than 2–3 weeks). Often, malignant ulcers are associated with tobacco and alcohol use. They are found predominantly in certain anatomical sites, with the tongue and floor of mouth being the commonest, followed by the retromolar region, tongue base and buccal mucosa. In recent years, there has been an increase in the proportion of Human Papilloma Virus-related (HPV-related) SCC of the oropharynx including the tonsil and tongue base areas. These tend to develop more posteriorly and inferiorly in the oropharynx (Fig 2.1).

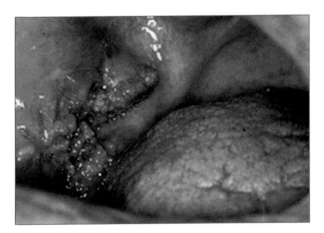

*Fig 2.1: Right tonsillar SCC secondary to chronic human papilloma virus infection.*

Benign mouth ulcers are, in general, painful. A painless ulcer is however extremely suspicious for malignancy and warrants an urgent cancer referral. Nevertheless, the presence of pain is not an entirely reassuring feature as malignant ulcers can also be painful, either in the early stages or at the outer margins of a large malignant ulcer (Fig 2.2). It is therefore very important to take a careful history of the ulcer's presentation and patient risk factors, as well as examining the oropharynx and neck thoroughly.

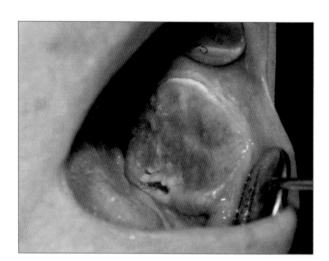

*Fig 2.2: This buccal mucosa SCC developed over months and despite its size was relatively asymptomatic.*

ORAL ULCERS

Malignant ulcers are often destructive, with migration of the ulcer beyond the epithelium into surrounding tissues (e.g. with muscle/fat/bone at the ulcer base). Destruction of nearby peripheral nerves leads to altered sensation in the region of the ulcer (hence a painless ulcer) and may lead to sensory or motor disturbance distal to the nerve lesion (e.g. tongue or lip numbness for example). Destruction of nearby dentoalveolar bone leads to unexplainably loose or missing teeth; an ulcer adjacent to isolated mobile teeth is highly worrying. Irregular shape and most importantly, induration (palpable firmness) should raise suspicion for malignancy, as should the presence of lymphadenopathy in association with a persistent ulcer.

ORAL ULCERS

## WARNING: ULCERS WITH AREAS OF EXPOSED BONE

*An ulcer extending down to bone with no identified cause should be treated suspiciously until proven otherwise. However, exposed jaw (mandible/maxilla) bone in the mouth commonly results from non-cancerous conditions such as:*

- *Recent dental extraction with delayed healing (with/without a painful 'dry socket', also known as alveolar osteitis) is common, especially in poorly controlled diabetic patients for example. Delayed mucosal/gingival healing without an obvious cause (acute infection) should raise suspicion of other pathology, including malignancy.*

- *Bisphosphonate related osteonecrosis of the jaw (BRONJ): this phenomenon, believed to result from impaired vascularity, is much commoner in those who have received or are receiving intravenous bisphosphonate treatment. Less commonly, BRONJ can result from oral bisphosphonate use and this should be borne in mind; a short-term 'drug holiday' (in liaison with the patient's oncologist/surgeon etc.) may be appropriate whist the problem is under investigation.*

- *Osteoradionecrosis (ORN) of the jaw: a common avascular sequel of radiotherapy in patients with previous/existing head and neck tumours. In this situation of exposed avascular bone, it may be difficult to discern a recurring/new malignant ulcer from one caused by ORN. Patients should therefore be referred for urgent assessment by their surgeon.*

*In the setting of BRONJ and ORN, elective dental extractions and any other surgical exposure of the jaw bone is generally avoided where feasible, so as to avoid creating a larger area of exposed avascular bone with impaired healing. Treatments provided by the OMFS team may include drug therapy (Pentoxyphylline, Vitamin E and antibiotics), hyperbaric oxygen (for ORN in particular) and surgical microvascular reconstruction. Meticulous oral hygiene (e.g. with regular periodontal scaling, brushing and antiseptic mouth rinse) is essential. The general dentist is usually closely involved and responsible for this component of their management.*

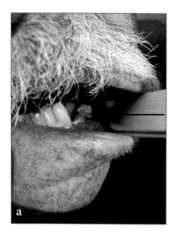 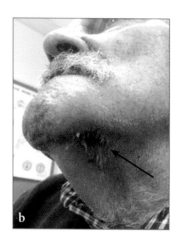

Fig 2.3: *This patient was suffering from BRONJ. Clinically the appearance of this necrotic ulcer with exposed bone (a) and involvement of the overlying skin with a sinus (b) is similar to that of an advanced oral cancer. However, elucidating the history of bisphosphonate use, along with a negative biopsy result is vital in guiding appropriate management.*

ORAL ULCERS

## ROUTINE REFERRAL

### PERSISTENT ULCERS

With persistent ulcers (especially single persistent ulcers), malignancy should be at the top of the differential diagnoses. However, in the absence of sinister features, other benign causes should also be considered. Benign persistent ulceration may be secondary to a persistent insult or irritation to the mucosa. This is commonly in the form of chronic local trauma: e.g. a traumatic ulcer secondary to the mucosa rubbing against a sharp tooth or dental filling (Fig 2.4), or application of topical irritants such as daily aspirin use (Fig 2.5). Furthermore, long-term systemic medications such as nicorandil can produce oral ulceration as a recognised side effect (Fig 2.6).

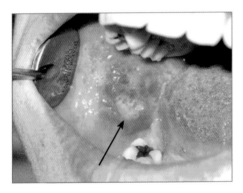

*Fig 2.4: Ulceration secondary to chronic dental trauma (cheek biting from unopposed/ laterally displaced upper molar teeth).*

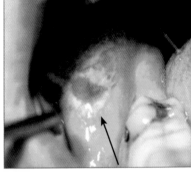

*Fig 2.5: Aspirin "burn" (irritation from prolonged chemical irritation of the mucosa). Note the surrounding mucosal changes.*

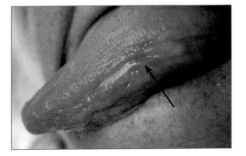

*Fig 2.6: Oral mucosal effects of long term nicorandil use: a shallow non-healing and very painful ulcer with no obvious traumatic cause.*

ORAL ULCERS

## RECURRENT ULCERS

In the absence of systemic disease, recurrent ulceration (often termed 'recurrent aphthous stomatitis' or RAS) is one of the commonest presentations and has affected up to 50% of the population at some stage or another. RAS generally presents in three clinical forms: major RAS (Fig 2.7) (a few large ulcers, more than 10mm in diameter, lasting weeks to months), minor RAS (Fig 2.8) (several small ulcers, less than 10mm in diameter, lasting 1–2 weeks) and herpetiform (Fig 2.9) (numerous pinhead-sized ulcers in crops, lasting 1–2 weeks).

ORAL ULCERS

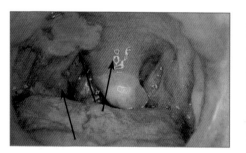

*Fig 2.7: Major aphthous ulceration.*

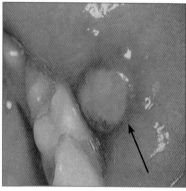

*Fig 2.8: Minor aphthous ulcer; note the red halo.*

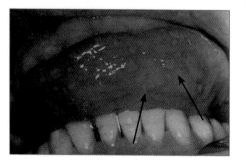

*Fig 2.9: Herpetiform ulceration*

Benign recurrent oral ulceration may be secondary to systemic autoimmune phenomena, including mucocutaneous conditions such as pemphigus (Fig 2.10), pemphigoid (Fig 2.11), Bechet's disease (Fig 2.12), erythema multiforme (Fig 2.13) and Stevens-Johnson syndrome (Fig 2.14). There are numerous mucocutaneous disorders to consider and an exhaustive list is beyond the scope of this book. However the presence of painful oral ulceration, with associated involvement of other mucosal or cutaneous surfaces should prompt an appropriate onward routine referral.

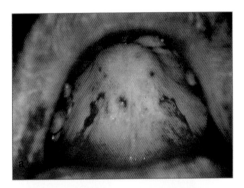

*Fig 2.10: Pemphigus of the oral mucosa; (a) of the palate, (b) of the buccal mucosa before and (c) after treatment with topical and oral steroids.*

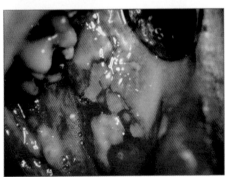

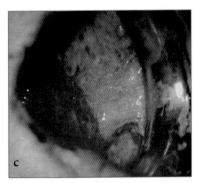

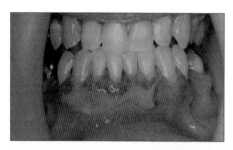

*Fig 2.11: Mucous membrane pemphigoid*

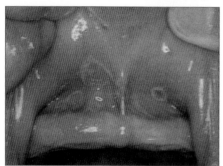

*Fig 2.12: Recurrent oral ulceration in a patient with Bechet's disease*

ORAL ULCERS

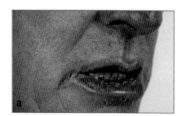

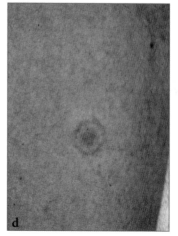

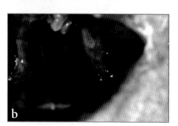

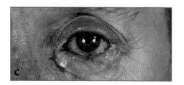

*Fig 2.13: Orofacial and cutaneous presentations of Erythema Multiforme involving the lips (a), the right buccal mucosa (b), the facial skin (c) and a peripheral target lesion (d).*

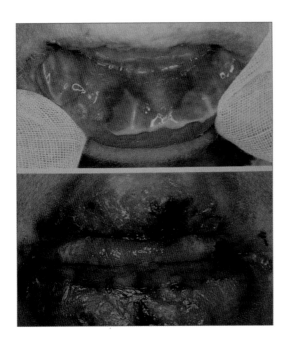

*Fig 2.14: Stevens Johnson syndrome*

Recurrent oral ulceration (with episodes of relapse and remission and/ or large ulcers) can be extremely debilitating to patients and warrants investigation and management in secondary care. Major RAS commonly requires topical and/or systemic immunosuppressive treatment for symptom management.

Minor RAS can be managed initially in primary care. Patients should be initially investigated for nutritional deficiency (haematinics and zinc levels should be evaluated) and stress; such causes should be managed as appropriate. Once the above are ruled out a simple trial of Benzydamine Hydrochloride (Difflam™) mouthwash with/without a steroid mouthwash (e.g. prednisolone or betamethasone) can be initiated. However, if symptom control is inadequate, or the underlying aetiology is unclear, routine referral to secondary care is warranted.

## REFERRAL TO DENTIST

If you have a strong suspicion based on the location and/or history that the ulcer is secondary to local trauma i.e. a sharp tooth, then the patient should see their own dentist in the first instance. However, in such a situation, it is important to liaise with the patient and follow up on the outcome to ensure that the lesion has indeed resolved. Any ulcer that persists despite appropriate measures should of course be referred via the urgent cancer route to secondary care for further assessment.

## MONITOR IN PRIMARY CARE

### SINGLE EPISODE OF ULCERATION

A single and completely resolved episode of ulceration does usually not warrant referral to secondary care and commonly results from local trauma, infection, stress or idiopathic causes. As long as there are no sinister features to cause concern, this can be safely monitored in primary care.

ORAL ULCERS

# CHAPTER 3: PATCHES ON THE ORAL MUCOSA

## INTRODUCTION

Patches on the oral mucosa are commonly seen in general practice. Unlike lumps, patches can be difficult to delineate and a single cause/type can be extremely heterogeneous in appearance: both in colour and morphology. Patches are commonly white, pigmented, red, or a mixture of colours. Even though initial treatment for patches of differing causes may be similar, the main message from this chapter is to be aware that certain types have a greater capacity for pre-malignancy and eventual malignant change or may even represent an early cancer.

The presence of particular sinister features (as discussed below) will direct towards a more urgent management approach. Their absence however will enable the Primary Care Clinician to methodically approach investigation and management.

Patches are often flat/macular in nature. Unlike lumps, they often do not have any unusual feel to them, and clinical diagnosis can be challenging, based on visual appearance alone. For this reason we divide our flowchart into patches that are 'mainly red', 'mainly white' or 'pigmented'. From this initial assessment you can then consider location, nearby structures and sinister features to arrive at the appropriate referral outcome.

Certain features in the history and clinical examination should immediately ring alarm bells. Risk factors (a smoking history and/or notable alcohol consumption) make premalignancy/malignancy a very real possibility. Lesion progression with induration and/or ulceration, altered sensation or lymphadenopathy makes malignant change an almost certainty, and would also warrant an urgent cancer referral.

**ASK:**

- Painful / painless?
- Bleeding?
- Duration (< / > 3 weeks?)
- Had similar problems before?
- Any skin diseases (e.g. lichen planus)
- Denture wearer?
- History of bruxism?
- Risk factor history

**LOOK:**

- Red / white / mixed / pigmented?
- Does the patch wipe off?
- Site, size, shape (irregular?), edge (well/poorly defined?)
- Local trauma (check denture / sharp teeth / cheek biting / dental filling)
- Is it soft or firm?
- Palpate for cervical lymphadenopathy

**SINISTER FEATURES:**

- Bleeding
- Lymphadenopathy
- Motor / sensory disturbance
- Rapid progression
- Red / mixed colouration
- Strong risk factor history
- Ulceration / induration of surrounding tissue

PATCHES ON THE
ORAL MUCOSA

# DO: MANAGEMENT ALGORITHM

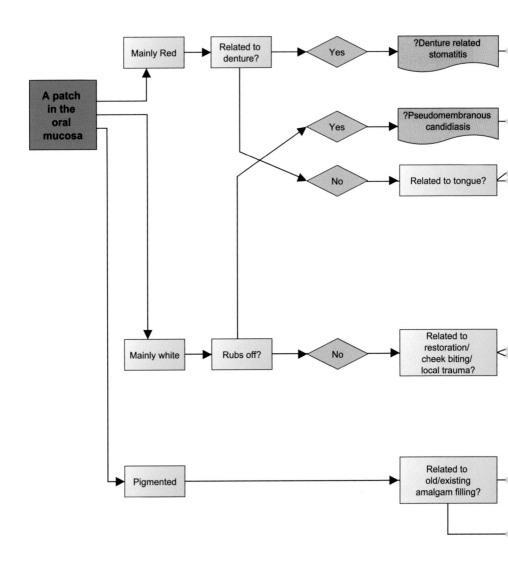

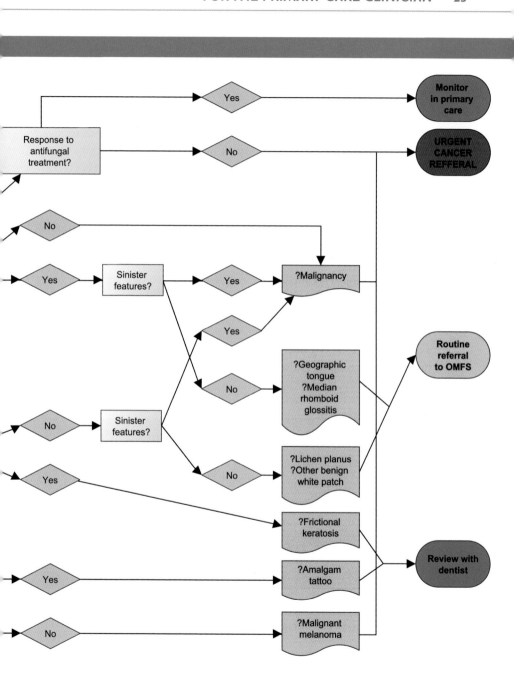

# URGENT CANCER REFERRAL

As mentioned earlier, red, white and pigmented patches can all represent sinister disease.

In general, redness indicates a degree of epithelial atrophy (which may eventually lead to erosion/ulceration). **A red/red-white patch of unknown origin (erythroplakia/erythroleukoplakia) is suspicious for premalignancy/malignant change and warrants urgent referral (Fig 3.1).**

A white patch that does not rub off gently with a tongue depressor or a damp gauze swab often indicates a 'thickening' of the epithelium, with an increased production of keratin. This keratosis may represent premalignant change and there should be a low threshold for onward referral as a potential cancer. When there is no identifiable cause, a tenacious white patch in the mouth is called leukoplakia and may well be a premalignant lesion. It may be homogenous or non-homogenous in appearance (Fig 3.2). Sublingual keratosis is also known as 'floor of mouth leukoplakia' and is a premalignant lesion associated with smoking. It has a characteristic 'ebbing tide' appearance (Fig 3.3). Syphilitic leukoplakia (usually of the tongue) is also premalignant.

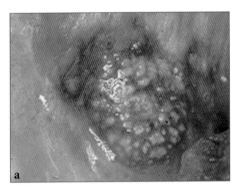 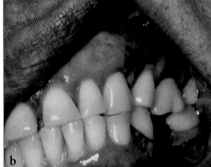

*Fig 3.1: Erythroleukoplakia (a) of the right buccal mucosa and (b) of the buccal gingiva in a patient with a history of oral submucous fibrosis.*

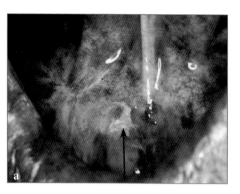

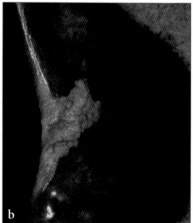

Fig 3.2: Leukoplakia: (a) of the floor of mouth, (b) classic homogenous type; involving the right oral comissure, (c) classic non-homogenous type; involving the buccal mucosa.

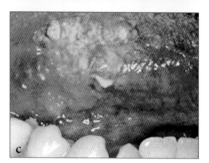

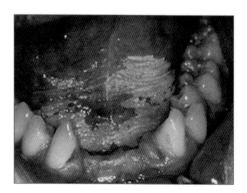

Fig 3.3: Sublingual keratosis; floor of mouth leukoplakia demonstrating the classic 'ebbing tide' appearance.

PATCHES ON THE ORAL MUCOSA

Oral submucous fibrosis is a premalignant condition associated with betel nut (paan) chewing; a habit common in, but not exclusive to, South Asian cultures. It presents with a pale, scarred appearance to the buccal mucosa, making it rigid and restricting mouth opening (see Chapter 7) (Fig 3.4).

Pigmented lesions tend to be blue or black in colour. Importantly, in the presence of sinister features and absence of an obvious cause, melanoma must be a consideration (Fig 3.5) and patients with such lesions should be referred urgently.

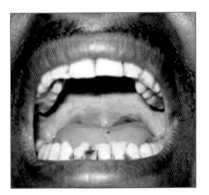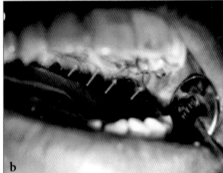

*Fig 3.4: Intraoral appearance of oral submucous fibrosis: note the pale scarred appearance (a) and web-like bands of scar tissue leaving abnormal rigidity to the mucosa on palpation and limitation in mouth opening (b). Malignant change (such as ulceration and/or colour change) may also be seen (arrows).*

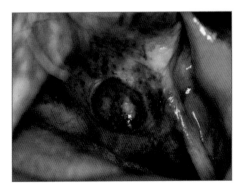

*Fig 3.5: Malignant melanoma of the palate.*

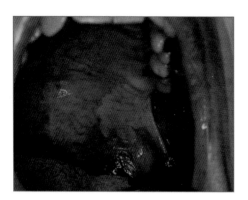

*Fig 3.6: Keratosis in the palate of a cigar smoker.*

It is important to note that it is not just the appearance of the lesion that is important, but also the site. For example, a flattened white/red patch in the palate in a cigar or reverse smoker is a premalignant lesion until proven otherwise (Fig 3.6). The tongue and floor of mouth are the two commonest sites for premalignant/malignant change and, based on probability alone, lesions in these locations should be managed with a high index of suspicion and referred appropriately.

Unfortunately the general appearance of a patch (red/white in colour) is not exclusive to any single cause. Some patches have a very heterogeneous appearance of atrophy (redness) and keratosis. Interestingly, candidiasis, premalignant change and lichen planus (in particular) can have a variety of clinical appearances and may change within days. Oral lichen planus (LP) typically (but not exclusively) presents with bilateral lesions on the mucosa/tongue/gingiva. Its appearance is highly variable and heterogeneous, and several subtypes have been described, the most common of which are the lace-like reticular form (Fig 3.7) and plaque-like (Fig 3.8) form. Patients may present with no symptoms, or experience soreness and discomfort in the area when eating/drinking certain foods (i.e. spicy food). As a Primary Care Clinician, it is important to understand that lesions with erosive or ulcerative characteristics have a higher potential for pre-malignancy (Fig 3.9).

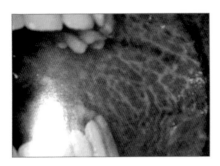

Fig 3.7: Reticular lichen planus of the buccal mucosa.

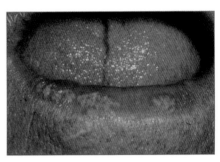

Fig 3.8: Plaques of oral lichen planus affecting the lip vermillion.

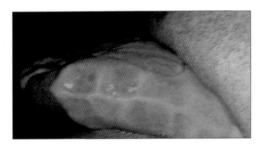

Fig 3.9: Longstanding erosive lichen planus of the anterior tongue; high capacity for malignant change.

If LP is suspected, it is important to check for involvement of other epithelial sites (eyes, skin, genital mucosa), which may point to a systemic condition requiring input from other specialties e.g. vulvovaginal LP. As mentioned, LP is thought by some to have premalignant potential. For this reason, it should be assessed at least once in secondary care and monitored actively for any suspicious changes in the long term. Most often an incisional biopsy will be performed. Treatment for LP ranges based upon disease severity from a simple steroid mouthwash and other topical applications, to systemic immunosuppressive medications.

Lichenoid reaction has a similar clinical and histopathological appearance to LP (although is commonly asymmetrically distributed in the mouth) but usually is secondary to outside causes (drugs, heavy metals or even a change in toothpaste). The aim of management is to identify and remove the offending cause, as well as relieving symptoms in a similar fashion to LP.

## ROUTINE REFERRAL

Many patches without sinister lesions may still require a biopsy to establish a diagnosis. However the decision to biopsy is often subjective and based upon the clinician's experience and the time course of the presentation. The decision to biopsy is best left to those in secondary care (it would be very unusual for a general medical practitioner to biopsy an oral lesion though some general dental practitioners do perform biopsies for presumed-benign lesions in dental practice), allowing an experienced clinician to examine the lesion in-situ, in its native environment beforehand. The Primary Care Clinician should however be aware and counsel their patient that this may be the first investigation once referred.

### RED PATCHES

Geographic tongue (also known as benign migratory glossitis) has a characteristic 'map-like' morphology, occurring on the dorsum of the tongue (Fig 3.10). Its cause is unknown and although it results in alternating areas of sore, red, atrophic mucosa, it is entirely benign and there is no known link with premalignancy or cancer. Diagnosis is made on clinical examination only. Nevertheless, should areas of atrophy fail to resolve within 3 weeks, and in the absence of sinister features, routine referral to the OMFS team is perfectly reasonable.

PATCHES ON THE ORAL MUCOSA

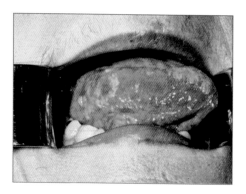

*Fig 3.10: Geographic tongue.*

## WHITE PATCHES

Candidal infection can result in a pseudo-membranous coating of the epithelial surface, leaving a white patch. A white patch that easily wipes off with a tongue depressor is highly suggestive of pseudomembranous candidiasis and should respond promptly and completely to antifungal treatments. It is often worth asking a patient if they are using a steroid inhaler or if they wear dentures (see page 34).

Another cause of a benign white patch is an inflammatory keratosis caused by drugs such as aspirin, which can 'burn' the epithelial in a similar fashion to mechanical trauma (See Chapter 2) (Fig 2.5, page 16). Lastly, confusingly, despite the name, hairy oral leukoplakia is not a premalignant lesion but is secondary to EBV infection and may be a presenting feature of HIV infection or immunosuppression (Fig 3.11).

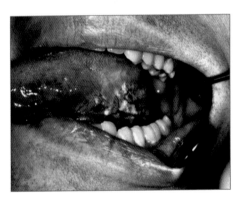

*Fig 3.11: Hairy oral leukoplakia in a patient with untreated HIV infection.*

## REFERRAL TO DENTIST

One of the commonest benign causes of a white patch in the mouth is frictional keratosis, where a thickening (and therefore whitening) of the epithelium occurs in reaction to chronic mechanical trauma including recurrent cheek biting. Consequently, a diagnosis of frictional keratosis should be made only if there is an obvious cause (i.e. a rough dental filling or a sharp tooth rubbing on the affected area, or a white thickening of the buccal mucosa in-line with the occlusal plane (the line of where the upper and lower teeth meet); sometimes described as a 'cheek-biting white patch' (Fig 3.12). Cheek biting is often bilateral. Nonetheless, in a smoker or even when there is any doubt, a biopsy is sometimes done to be completely sure, especially if there is no evidence of trauma

Pigmented (blue/brown) lesions in the mouth are common and often arise through 'tattooing' of the mucosa from an existing or previous amalgam dental filling (Fig 3.13).

PATCHES ON THE ORAL MUCOSA

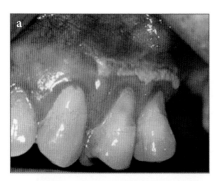

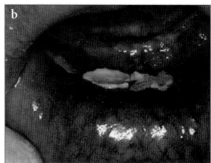

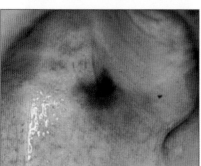

*Fig 3.12: (a) Frictional keratosis from overzealous toothbrushing and (b) a poorly fitting denture.*

*Fig 3.13: Amalgam tattoo; unchanging pigmentation adjacent to a site of a previous longstanding amalgam dental filling (unlike malignant melanoma – cf. Fig 3.5, page 28).*

## MONITOR IN PRIMARY CARE

Several conditions can safely be monitored in the primary care setting. The first are red atrophic changes commonly related to an underlying infection such as oral candidiasis particularly seen in denture-wearers. These patients commonly suffer from denture-related stomatitis as a result of inadequate hygiene and simple treatment with improved denture hygiene, topical and/or oral antifungals can resolve the situation within days (Fig 3.14). The clinical picture is of a red patch confined to the mucosa that is in direct contact with the underside of the denture. Patients may often have angular cheilitis as well, which can be sore, and which they describe as a sore red area that doesn't heal. Similarly candida infection of the tongue can present with a classical midline red patch on the dorsum of the tongue, known as median rhomboid glossitis (Fig 3.15). Where the red patch clinically appears to be typical of candidiasis and lacking any sinister features in the presentation, a short period of treatment with topical and/or systemic antifungal treatment combined with active monitoring is appropriate. However, should atrophic candida infections fail to resolve with appropriate treatment, erythroplakia (and therefore premalignancy) remains to be a high possibility, warranting urgent referral.

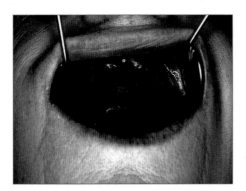

*Fig 3.14: "Denture-related stomatitis".*

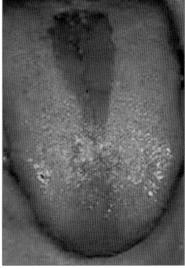

*Fig 3.15: Median rhomboid glossitis.*

PATCHES ON THE ORAL MUCOSA

White patches can be a completely physiological phenomenon, such as Fordyce spots (Fig 3.16) and leukoedema; a bluish/white hue of the mucosa, more commonly found in people with darker skin pigmentation. Whilst benign, these lesions may be difficult for a practitioner in primary care to confidently diagnose. Therefore, it is acceptable to make a routine referral to OMFS, should any doubt regarding the diagnosis exist.

A common cause of a brown midline patch of the tongue is 'black hairy tongue' (Fig 3.17). This in itself is a benign condition of filiform papillae (taste buds) overgrowth, trapping pigments from food, bacteria and yeast. It is usually of no significance, but may be a presenting feature of HIV infection or immunosuppression.

*Fig 3.16: Fordyce spots of the buccal mucosa.*

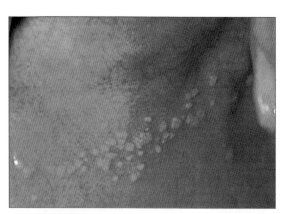

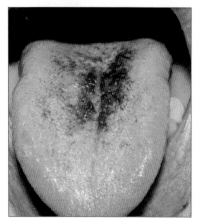

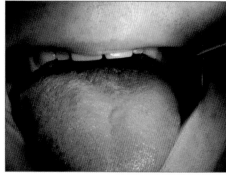

*Fig 3.17: Black hairy tongue.*

PATCHES ON THE ORAL MUCOSA

# CHAPTER 4: LUMPS IN THE MOUTH

## INTRODUCTION

The mouth is composed of numerous tissue types, located to specific sites. As such, the nature of a lump in the mouth is often dependent upon its anatomical location. For example, odontogenic tumours and cysts (i.e. of dental origin) are in general limited to the tooth-bearing regions. Benign salivary swellings are commoner in the floor of mouth where both major and minor salivary glands are plentiful. Malignancy can occur anywhere within the mouth, but primary SCC is commoner in certain high-risk sites.

Lumps in the mouth are usually abnormal. As a result, almost all lumps require management in secondary care or in some cases primary dental care (if of a simple dental nature). A reasonable differential diagnosis can be achieved by its **anatomical location** and this is the first question that our referral flowchart-algorithm asks. After this we focus on consistency (hard/soft) and the presence of sinister features. Getting the actual diagnosis is not essential (routine OMFS referral for biopsy and/or other investigations will suffice), but identifying a lump suspicious for malignancy is. Certain features in the history and clinical examination should ring alarm bells and these are highlighted in the 'sinister features' box. Their absence however will enable the Primary Care Clinician to rationally take a stepwise routine approach to investigation and management.

## ASK:

- Risk factor assessment
- Painful vs painless
- Duration (< / > 3 weeks?)
- Previous history of oral cancer
- Other associated orofacial symptoms?
- Does it swell on eating?
- Discharge in the mouth
- Any swelling in the neck (submandibular gland)?
- PMHx of autoimmune diseases?

## LOOK:

- Site (e.g. tongue, retromolar, attached gingiva, floor of mouth)? Tissue layer?
- Size
- Features – shape, colour (e.g. vascular?), edge
- Fluctuance?
- Nearby teeth deviated? Loose?
- Palpate for lymphadenopathy

## SINISTER FEATURES:

- A lump in the upper lip and soft palate is malignant until proven otherwise
- Associated ulceration
- Fixity to deep tissues
- Irregular border
- Lymphadenopathy
- Nerve weakness/altered sensation of the tongue or lip/cheek
- On high risk areas (lateral tongue, floor of mouth, retromolar)
- Previous oral cancer
- Rapidly growing
- Strong risk factor history (smoking, alcohol, betel nut chewing)

LUMPS IN THE MOUTH

# DO: MANAGEMENT ALGORITHM

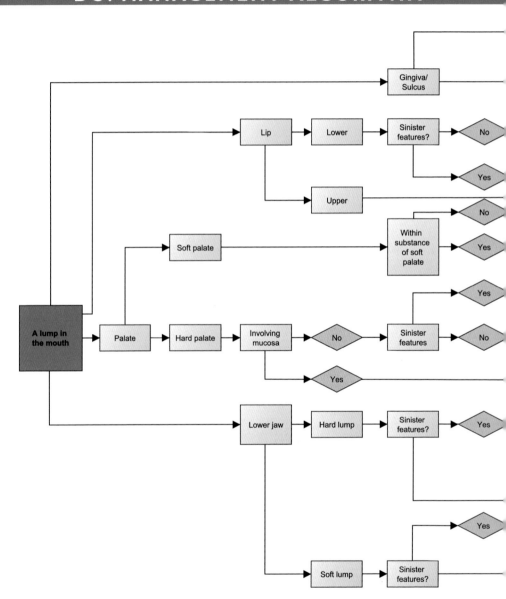

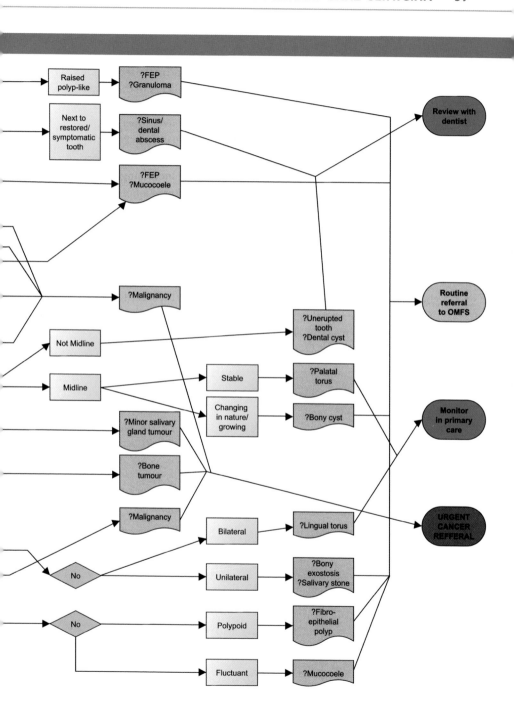

**LUMPS IN THE MOUTH**

# URGENT CANCER REFERRAL

The mouth can be the site of numerous types of primary malignancy. Of these, SCC is the commonest (up to 95% of all cancers in the mouth). SCC (discussed in Chapter 2) typically presents as a non-healing ulcer which then becomes indurated and fixed to underlying structures, eventually taking on the form of a 'lump' (which can be very hard in consistency when bone is involved). Patients commonly have a history of tobacco smoking and excess alcohol consumption but an increasing proportion of patients are now presenting without a significant alcohol or smoking history, thought to relate to the increasing incidence of Human Papilloma Virus (HPV) related SCC. However, the clinical appearance can be entirely variable, with only a small ulcer or other minor mucosal changes. Therefore, it is important to be aware of any sinister features and/or risk factors in the presentation, regardless of whether or not the lump has the hallmarks of a 'classic' SCC. By frequency, high-risk areas for primary oral SCC include the lateral border of the tongue, the floor of mouth and the retromolar regions (Figs. 4.1–4.3).

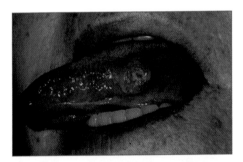

*Fig 4.1: SCC left lateral border of tongue*

*Fig 4.2: SCC Floor of mouth (lower left)*

*Fig 4.3: SCC left retromolar region*

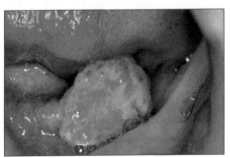

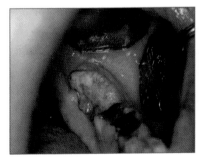

Salivary gland malignancy is fairly common. The site of presentation does have a significant influence on the likelihood of a salivary tumour being malignant, with a general point to remember that **the smaller the gland, the greater the chance of malignancy.** Also lumps of the upper lip and junction of hard and soft palate are always taken seriously and are malignant until proven otherwise (Fig 4.4). Malignant salivary gland tumours of major glands (parotid, submandibular and sublingual) may simply present as a gradual and progressive swelling of the gland, which may eventually lead to an indurated texture on bimanual palpation. Involvement of nearby motor and sensory nerves leads to motor deficits (facial nerve in parotid malignancy, hypoglossal and/or lingual nerve in submandibular malignancy). Involvement of the salivary ducts causes obstructive symptoms (which, importantly to note, are common with benign salivary disorders as well).

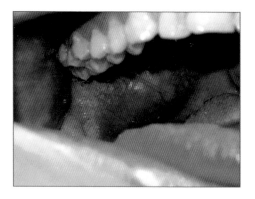

*Fig 4.4: A suspicious tumour of the soft/hard palate junction: most likely a malignant salivary neoplasm until proven otherwise.*

LUMPS IN THE MOUTH

Fortunately, tumours of the parotid and submandibular glands are more commonly benign (80% and 60% respectively) while about 50% of sublingual gland tumours are malignant. Benign tumours are typically slow growing and discrete (Fig 4.5). As mentioned above, solid minor salivary gland tumours of the palate on the other hand are almost always malignant, typically presenting as a progressive indurated swelling (with/without other sinister features such as lymphadenopathy) (Figs. 4.6 and 4.7).

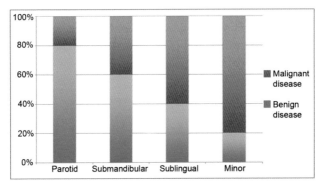

Fig 4.5: Frequency of malignant vs benign disease as the size of salivary gland gets smaller

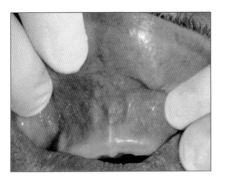

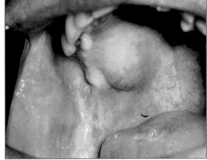

Fig 4.6: Minor salivary gland tumour in the upper lip – firm not cystic

Fig 4.7: Suspected tumour at junction of hard and soft palate

Malignant bone tumours may be primary or secondary/metastatic in origin. SCCs occurring in the mucosa commonly spread to underlying jaw bones causing bony deformity, tooth mobility/loss and peripheral neuropathy to any nerves running through the medullary bone (e.g. chin numbness due to inferior alveolar nerve compression from an expanding mandibular tumour). The common malignant tumours that metastasise to bone (breast, lung, prostate) can of course have jaw metastases. Rarely, malignant primary bone tumours may be odontogenic (from tooth tissue) in origin, such as ameloblastic carcinoma, though these are very rare in comparison to SCC (see glossary). Differentiating these from simple odontogenic cysts and tumours can be very challenging, even after biopsy and histological examination. The underlying diagnosis is therefore not so important, but identifying bony swellings with sinister features that warrant urgent assessment in secondary care, is.

Hard and soft tissue sarcomas of the orofacial region are very rare but take on some of the hallmark features of other primary malignancies (like SCC). A progressively expanding mass of clinically unclear aetiology should raise concern of this possible diagnosis.

## REFERRAL TO DENTIST

Infected teeth often lead to periapical (tip of the root) abscess formation, which in turn can track along the path of least resistance to the gingival surface. This presents as a dental sinus or 'gum boil' (Fig 4.8). Teeth with associated periapical infection may have a preceding history of dental pain / symptoms and will be tender to percussion (tapping). They warrant referral to a dentist for prompt attention.

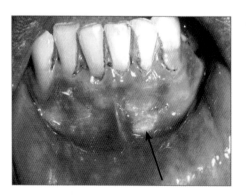

*Fig 4.8: Discharging sinus from anterior teeth into buccal sulcus*

LUMPS IN THE MOUTH

### IMMEDIATE REFERRAL

Sometimes however, instead of erupting on the gingival surface, abscesses can track into fascial spaces of the neck causing formation of large (and at times airway compromising) abscesses or a Ludwig's angina (floor-of-mouth cellulitis with severe sequelae of airway compromise) (Figs. 4.9–4.12). Figure 4.12 illustrates the common routes of fascial spread of dental sepsis.

Small mouth swellings thought to be infective (i.e. a buccal sulcus abscess) require urgent attention by a dentist. Larger neck space swellings, or if the patient has any signs of impending airway obstruction (raised floor-of-mouth, difficulty swallowing, hoarseness of voice), facial cellulitis (placing the patient at risk of periorbital cellulitis and cavernous sinus thrombosis) or systemic compromise / sepsis, should be referred immediately to the on-call OMFS team. **If you see an acute patient who is drooling and cannot swallow saliva, with facial swelling, then dial emergency services as this is a sign of impending airway obstruction.**

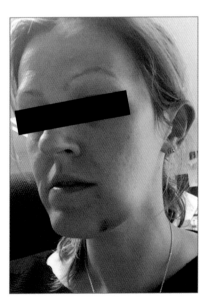

*Fig 4.9: This buccal space abscess was secondary to an infected osteosynthesis plate but the appearance is also classical of dentoalveolar infection.*

LUMPS IN THE MOUTH

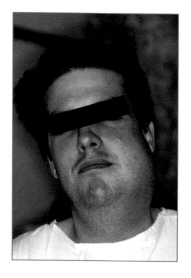
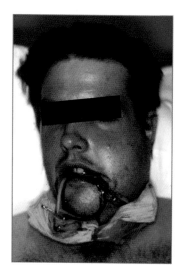

Fig 4.10: Neck space (submandibular) abscess with an accompanying Ludwig's Angina (floor of mouth cellulitis), resulting in acute airway compromise. This patient required emergency incision and drainage (via both neck and intraoral incisions) as well as extraction of causative teeth to prevent further airway obstruction.

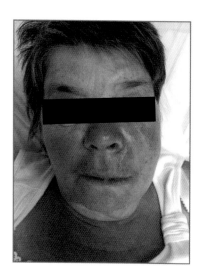

Fig 4.11: Canine space/fossa abscess; a para-nasal swelling extending vertically upwards towards the eye, putting the patient at risk of orbital cellulitis (and potentially cavernous sinus thrombosis) if left untreated.

LUMPS IN THE MOUTH

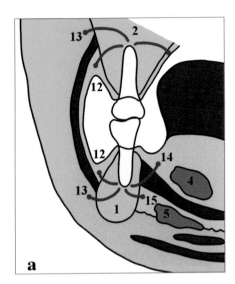

a

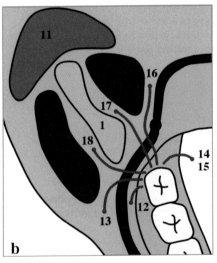

b

*Fig 4.12. (a) coronal section of cheek and oral cavity, and (b) transverse section at the level of the occlusal plane, to show the routes of spread of dental sepsis.*

1. Mandible
2. Maxilla
3. Tongue
4. Sublingual gland
5. Submandibular gland
6. Mylohyoid
7. Buccinator
8. Superior constrictor
9. Medial pterygoid
10. Masseter
11. Parotid gland
12. **Buccal sulcus**
13. **Buccal space**
14. **Sublingual space**
15. **Submandibular space**
16. **Parapharyngeal space**
17. **Pterygomandibular space**
18. **Submasseteric space**

## ROUTINE REFERRAL

In the absence of an obvious dental infection, a fleshy mobile lump on the gingiva or mucosa is commonly a fibroepithelial polyp (Fig 4.13). If cystic (and classically on the mucosa of the lower lip or floor of mouth), a salivary mucocoele of a minor salivary gland is a likely possibility (Fig 4.14). A mucocoele is a collection of saliva extruding from a salivary gland into surrounding connective tissues. A ranula is a generally larger mucocoele of the floor-of-mouth and by definition arises from a sublingual gland (Fig 4.15). Mucocoeles are generally harmless but can become infected and can also be a nuisance to patients, especially as they expand to become very large. These can therefore be referred as routine to OMFS for excision. As mentioned previously, upper lip lumps are taken very seriously.

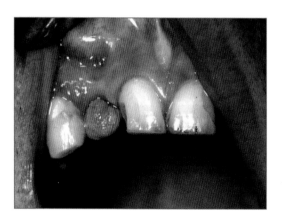

*Fig 4.13: Fibroepithelial polyp from an inflammed right upper lateral incisor tooth socket*

LUMPS IN THE MOUTH

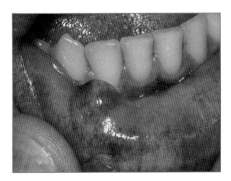

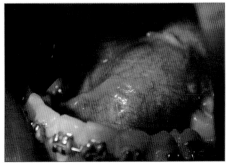

Fig 4.14: Mucocoele of the lower lip          Fig 4.15: Ranula

LUMPS IN THE
MOUTH

A hard lump of the mandible or maxilla is most commonly a 'torus'. These are simple physiological bony outgrowths (exostoses) of indefinite duration (for as long as the patient can remember) usually found as either a symmetrical smooth midline swelling of the hard palate, or bilateral symmetrical smooth swellings of the mandible (classically on the lingual/inside surface) (Fig 4.16 and 4.17). Without any sinister features or ambiguity over the clinical diagnosis, these lesions can be monitored safely in primary care. Needless to say, any subsequent change or progression of such a swelling warrants a referral to secondary care. Sometimes a salivary stone from the sublingual gland can sit in the floor of the mouth and mimic a mandibular torus. In the presence of any salivary symptoms a routine referral is indicated.

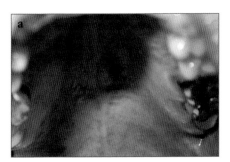

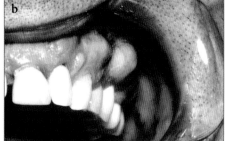

Fig 4.16: Palatal torus (a) and maxillary tori (b)

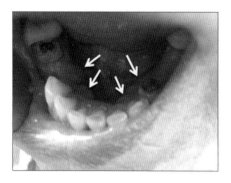

*Fig 4.17: Lingual tori (highlighted with white arrows): bilateral symmetrical bony swellings on the lingual aspect of the mandible. Classically they will have been present for as long as the patient can remember (i.e. not a noticeably new swelling for the patient but may become increasingly uncomfortable with time).*

Benign bone cysts and tumours of the jaws are commonly seen in the OMFS department. Often, these hard bony swellings are odontogenic in origin and relate to either teeth (infected or unerupted teeth for example), dental embryological tissue, giant cell granuloma or may arise from the bone itself (as elsewhere in the body). Cysts and benign swellings (i.e. slowly developing swellings in the absence of cancer risk factors or sinister features) should be routinely referred as with time they may expand and become very destructive to the surrounding tissues, as seen in ameloblastoma (Fig 4.18).

LUMPS IN THE MOUTH

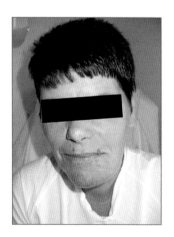
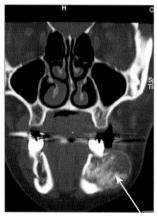

*Fig 4.18: This patient presented with a hard painless swelling fixed to the left mandible. CT revealed a mixed-density tumour with expansion of the buccal cortex. Enucleation of the lesion was performed and it was found to be a cementoblastoma; a benign odontogenic tumour of the supportive/periodontal tissues.*

# CHAPTER 5: LUMPS OF THE FACE

## INTRODUCTION

There are many causes of lumps on the face and they can present a significant diagnostic challenge. Furthermore, there is considerable cross over between skin tumours and swellings of subcutaneous tissue origin. As with all lumps and bumps, a history and clinical examination is paramount in helping to differentiate benign from malignant pathology.

While the presence of sinister features, as discussed below, should prompt urgent management approaches, their absence still requires a rational approach to investigation, management and referral if required.

To simplify management, the first question the algorithm asks is to divide lumps into those within the skin and those deep to the skin surface. You can then consider if it is a hard or soft lump, and if there are signs of infection or whether you consider it to be sinister. This stepwise approach should facilitate the appropriate referral outcome.

**ASK:**

- How long?
- Getting worse?
- Painful?
- Any previous infection or discharge?
- Previous facial trauma?
- Aesthetic concerns?
- Associated symptoms?
- If in region of parotid – mealtime symptoms?

**LOOK:**

- Site and size – where is it on the face? What tissue layer?
- Shape, surface and edge – smooth or irregular?
- Colour
- Consistency – Soft vs hard – (bony hard suggests osteoma/bone pathology)
- Fluctuance
- Attached to skin/deep tissue?
- Signs of infection?
- Palpate for cervical lymphadenopathy

**SINISTER FEATURES:**

- Fixity to underlying structures
- Irregular border
- Lymphadenopathy
- Multiple pigmentations
- Nerve involvement (altered sensation or weakness)
- Rapidly increasing in size
- Ulceration/bleeding

LUMPS OF THE FACE

# DO: MANAGEMENT ALGORITHM

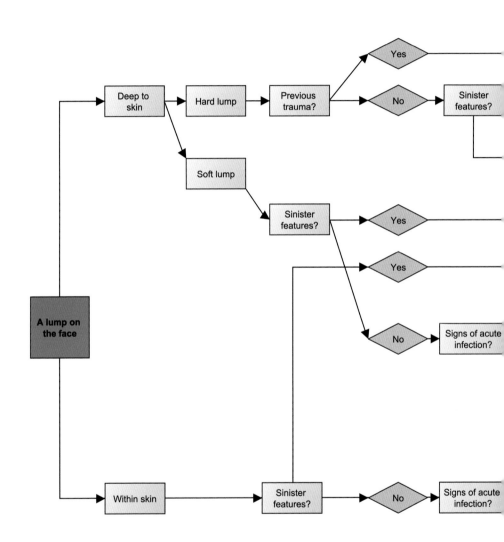

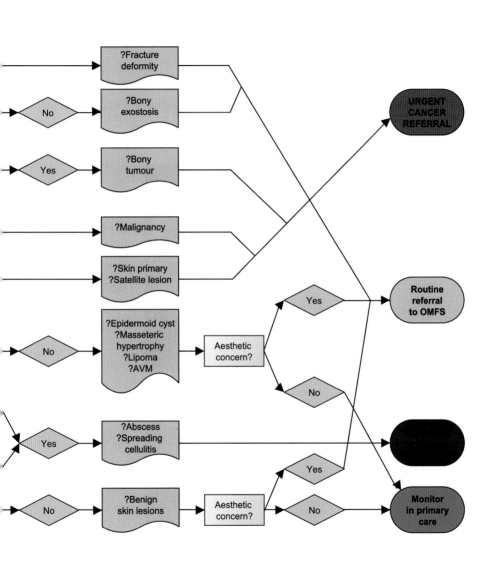

## URGENT CANCER REFERRAL

Typical malignant lesions you might encounter would include skin cancers, other soft tissue cancers and bony tumours (the latter are relatively rare). The presence of any sinister features would warrant an urgent referral to OMFS cancer services for assessment at a specialist unit.

You should be familiar with the assessment of facial skin cancers: basal cell carcinomas, squamous cell carcinomas and malignant melanomas (so these are purposely not discussed in detail) (Figs. 5.1–5.3). It is important

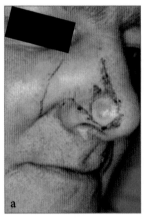
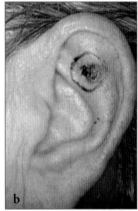

*Fig 5.1(a)BCC right nose with markings for surgical excision margin and local flap reconstruction.*

*Fig 5.1(b) BCC left pinna*

*Fig 5.1(c) BCC right forehead*

a

b

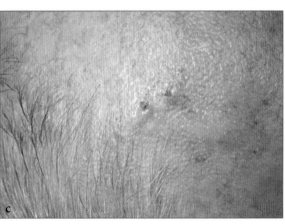

c

LUMPS OF THE FACE

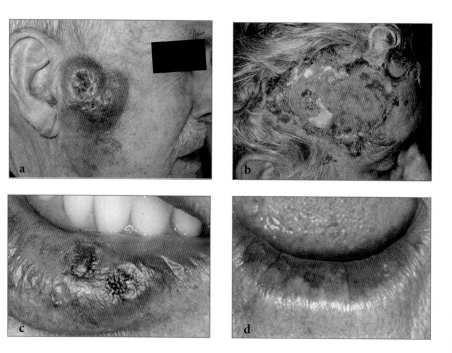

Fig 5.2(a) SCC right preauricular region

Fig 5.2 (b) Untreated large invasive SCC

Fig 5.2 (c) SCC of the lower lip

Fig 5.2 (d) Actinic keratosis of the lower lip is difficult to discern from SCC clinically and requires biopsy for differentiation. Note however that actinic keratosis is a premalignant lesion.

LUMPS OF THE FACE

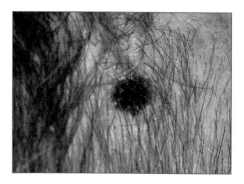

Fig 5.3: Malignant melanoma of the temple (Note: differential pigmentation and irregular border)

to instigate a prompt referral along the recognised cancer pathway, either to Dermatology, ENT or OMFS to ensure that these lesions can be given a definitive histological diagnosis and an appropriate management plan determined in the multi-disciplinary setting. This process will also be important to exclude potential malignancy – benign keratoacanthoma (KA) mimics squamous cell carcinoma in appearance, so should be referred for diagnostic purposes to avoid missing potentially malignant disease (Fig 5.4). Management of skin cancers can vary and includes topical chemotherapy, simple curettage under local anaesthesia, cryotherapy, laser therapy, Mohs micrographic surgery with appropriate reconstruction postoperatively as well as traditional excision surgery and radiotherapy.

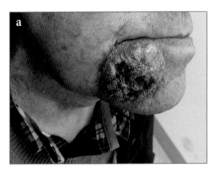 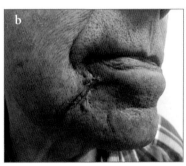

*Fig 5.4 (a) and (b): Keratoacanthoma (KA): This patient presented with a large ulcerative swelling with a necrotic centre. Malignancy was high on the list of differential diagnoses but a biopsy suggested KA. Watchful waiting by the maxillofacial team allowed this lesion to spontaneously regress, thus avoiding excisional surgery (which in comparison, with even the best reconstructive techniques, would have caused significant aesthetic compromise). Images courtesy of Mr Sankar Ananth and Mr Madhav Kittur, Morriston Hospital, Swansea, UK.*

Soft tissue malignancy, such as sarcomas originating from the head and neck region, are rare and therefore can be difficult to diagnose, let alone treat, so it is imperative that onward referral occurs at the earliest opportunity. A painless, soft mass with associated facial deformity is the commonest presentation and certainly the presence of accompanying sinister symptoms including visual disturbances, otalgia, sinus disease, facial weakness or sensory disturbance should increase the index of suspicion exponentially (Fig 5.5).

Bony growths will present with hard lumps that can be palpated around the facial skeleton. Such lumps can be related to the mandible, maxilla, frontal, nasal or temporal structures and while not all will be rapidly growing, the presence of any sinister features should again prompt urgent referral. It is important to assess the oral cavity as well, as lumps in the maxilla and mandible may be palpated intra-orally, can lead to movement or mobility/ loss of teeth and alteration to intraoral sensation.

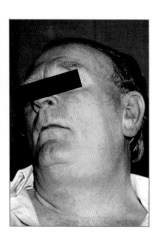
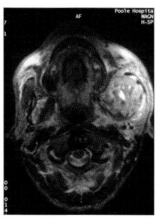

*Fig 5.5: A large tumour arising from the infratemporal/ pterygoid fossa with facial swelling. Differential diagnosis would include malignant parotid tumour, sarcoma, local or distant metastatic tumour.*

LUMPS OF THE FACE

# ROUTINE REFERRAL TO OMFS

The absence of sinister features can leave the clinician facing a wide range of potential differential diagnoses. Skin and deeper soft lumps are often a cause of functional or aesthetic concern, and should be referred for assessment and intervention. The Primary Care Clinician will commonly encounter epidermoid ("sebaceous") cysts and lipomas. Those that are problematic in terms of previous infection, interference with normal function or aesthetic concerns are often amenable to excision under local anaesthetic after routine referral to OMFS.

Other soft tissue lumps that are amenable to management in secondary care include masseteric hypertrophy, which occurs either in conjunction with or distinctly from TMJ symptoms. As such, it is again important to assess these cases in the full clinical context. Management can be conservative – soft diet, stress-relieving actions, or referral to a dental practitioner for construction of bite guards to be worn at night. If resistant to simple treatments, masseteric hypertrophy can respond well to regular Botulinum toxin injections, performed in secondary care.

The face is an extremely vascular part of the body. As such, arteriovenous anomalies are reasonably common, either in isolation or as part of a systemic phenomenon/syndrome. Commonly, these lesions are investigated by the OMFS team, using ultrasonography, MRI and/or CT imaging. It is important to rule out any intracranial extension (which if present, may put the patient at risk of catastrophic spontaneous intracranial haemorrhage). Treatment depends on cause and may be very simple (small strawberry naevi in young children often resolve following a period of active monitoring) (Fig 5.6). Some lesions respond to beta-blockers (propranolol), whereas others may require cryotherapy, sclerotherapy and interventional radiology with/without surgical excision (with associated risks of intraoperative bleeding) (Fig 5.7).

There are a number of hard tissue or bony lumps that can be referred routinely to the OMFS team. These would typically include bony exostoses, for example forehead osteomas (Fig 5.8). These can have social impacts for patients, who are often keen for them to be removed.

LUMPS OF THE FACE

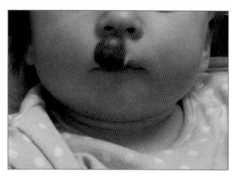

Fig 5.6: A haemangioma ('Strawberry Naevus') in a neonate; likely to regress completely through childhood. Image courtesy of Mr Andrew Monaghan, Queen Elizabeth Hospital, Birmingham, UK.

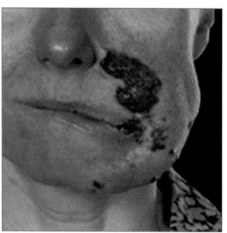

Fig 5.7: A large arteriovenous malformation. Image courtesy of Mr Andrew Monaghan, Queen Elizabeth Hospital, Birmingham, UK.

LUMPS OF THE FACE

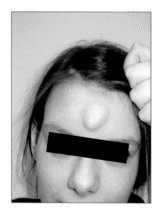
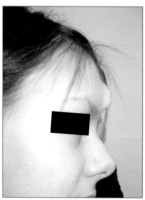

Fig 5.8: Frontal (forehead) osteoma.

Post-traumatic deformities are essentially a consequence of untreated or incompletely treated facial trauma resulting in bony healing of fracture components in incorrect/unreduced positions. These will result in facial asymmetry, bony prominences or patients reporting that they 'just look different'. A history of trauma (both treated and untreated) is paramount and should lead to the diagnosis. Patients with these deformities will warrant routine referral to an OMFS unit for a full assessment with 3-dimensional imaging. Surgical management may be complex, involving camouflage techniques, surgical intervention and psychological support.

## IMMEDIATE REFERRAL TO ON-CALL OMFS

Any soft tissue lumps in the face which appear infective (increasing pain, overlying erythema, systemic inflammatory response) can be discussed with and/or referred to the local on-call OMF surgeon. Such cases may require admission for antibiotic therapy or surgical drainage. Epidermoid ('sebaceous') cysts are the typical lesions on the face to become infected.

With acute onset infective swellings of the face, the most common cause is dental infection. A dental abscess arising from the upper canine teeth will present as canine fossa / infraorbital swellings (Fig 4.11), while teeth positioned more distally (posteriorly) in the dental arch will present with buccal space / cheek swellings (Fig 4.9). As such, the dentition should be carefully looked at in patients presenting with these signs. While the oral cavity may sometimes be less familiar to Primary Care Clinicians (including general medical practitioners), spreading sepsis and systemic symptoms will provide the most important information to help decide whether a patient requires referral for hospital management or can be referred to a local dentist for assessment. *Please refer to Chapter 4 for more information on dental sepsis and development of orofacial abscesses.*

## MONITOR IN PRIMARY CARE

Any lump on the face, which does not present with sinister features and does not present functional or aesthetic concerns can be safely monitored in primary care. However, it should be noted that regular review of these cases should be undertaken so any change or progression in symptoms can be noted and duly referred.

LUMPS OF THE FACE

## INTRODUCTION

A patient presenting with facial pain or altered sensation can be extremely difficult to diagnose and treat. Whilst organic causes may be obvious and can be treated accordingly, often there is a strong psychological component that can be difficult to overcome. For such a complex topic, the management algorithm overleaf may appear somewhat simple, but this is deliberate to keep the referral pathways clear.

Dental pathology is the commonest cause for facial pain and close liaison with the patient's dentist is invaluable. However, you should ideally have an understanding of all important causes (benign and malignant) that can be treated or referred appropriately. The first question in the management algorithm asks about the nature of the pain, as this feature will (most of the time) separate urgent cancer and routine referrals. If the pain is not characteristic of dental causes (and no sinister features are identified) then further decision needs to be made as to whether it is likely neuropathic, jaw joint related or non-specific (and therefore possibly psychological).

**ASK:**
- What is the problem: pain / paraesthesia / both?
- Pain history
  - Site – e.g. TMJ / trigeminal division?
  - Onset – e.g. sudden / gradual?
  - Character – e.g. sharp / dull / electric-shock like?
  - Radiation – e.g. to throat / ear etc.?
  - Associated symptoms – e.g. restricted jaw movements / speech / swallow?
  - Timing – constant / lasts for seconds?
  - Exacerbating / relieving factors – cold air / warmth / improves through the day etc.?
  - Severity (score out of 10)

- Progressively worse / fluctuating?
- History of dental problems in region of pain?
- History of pain syndromes, neurological disease (e.g. MS), psychological problems?
- Which medications have helped?

## LOOK:

- Any obvious facial or intraoral abnormalities / swellings etc.?
- Cranial nerves intact?
- Tenderness in region of the pain or not?
- Tenderness on firm palpation / pain on swallowing or eating / hyperaesthesia?
- Palpate for cervical lymphadenopathy

## SINISTER FEATURES:

- Associated swellings / oral ulceration
- Lymphadenopathy
- Oro-facial weakness / other cranial nerve motor deficit
- Paraesthesia or anaesthesia in a nerve distributuon
- Progressive trismus
- Rapidly progressive symptoms
- Visual / hearing disturbance

FACIAL PAIN / ALTERED SENSATION

# DO: MANAGEMENT ALGORITHM

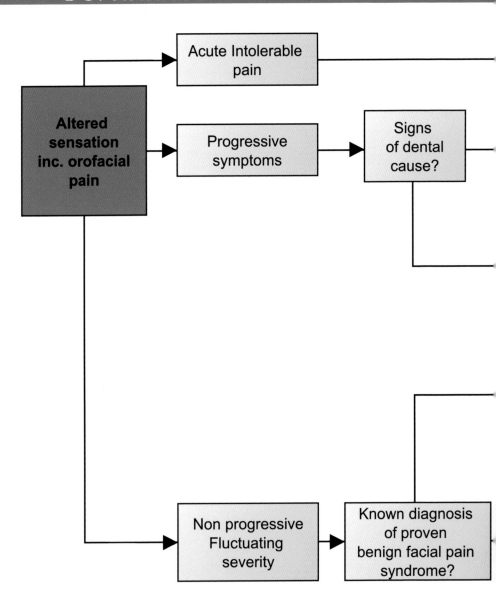

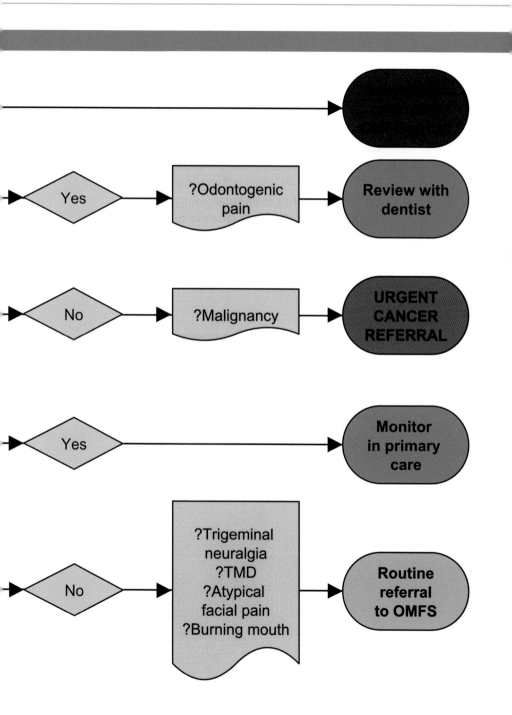

# URGENT CANCER REFERRAL

## FACIAL PAIN/ALTERED SENSATION OF MALIGNANCY

When considering facial pain or altered sensation associated with malignancy it is unlikely that this will be the only symptom. As described in the sinister features box, by the time these symptoms are present there will usually be other clinical signs that point towards a malignant cause and trigger an urgent cancer referral. The character of pain or altered sensation will vary according to the underlying malignant pathology. Therefore, facial pain and altered sensation associated with a mass or swelling is covered in detail elsewhere in this book. Progressive symptoms of pain, with any of the sinister features listed should prompt an urgent referral.

# ROUTINE REFERRAL

## BENIGN FACIAL PAIN SYNDROMES

Unfortunately this list is extensive. Below we discuss the common causes that a Primary Care Clinician should be aware of when making a routine referral. The many complex and rare causes not discussed will be identified in secondary care.

FACIAL PAIN / ALTERED SENSATION

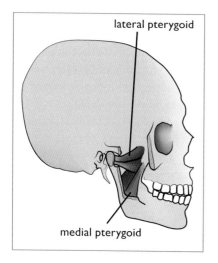 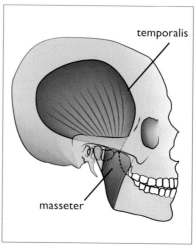

*Fig 6.1: TMJ showing the relevant muscles of mastication*

## TEMPOROMANDIBULAR DISORDER

Temporomandibular disorder (TMD) is an umbrella term describing dysfunction of the temporomandibular joint and associated muscular apparatus that causes pain and symptoms (Fig 6.1). Three diagnostic groups are acknowledged: muscle disorders, joint disc displacement and true TM joint arthritis. Causes include trauma, bruxism (teeth clenching), altered or malocclusion and disc and/or joint disease.

The dull aching pain of TMD may or may not be localised to the TM joint. Common symptoms are a 'noisy' or 'clicking' jaw caused by displacement of the joint disc or limited mouth opening due to disc displacement and/ or muscular spasm. It is important to appreciate however that jaw clicking (secondary to an anteriorly displaced disc) occurs in approximately one-third of the population. Otalgia, headache, pain behind the eye, neck stiffness and dizziness may accompany TMD. Palpation of the joint and muscles of mastication will elicit tenderness.

FACIAL PAIN /
ALTERED SENSATION

The treatment of these patients is to try to break the cycle of pain, causing muscle spasm and limited mouth opening and further pain, etc. In addition, efforts to address the psychological component that accompanies this chronic pain syndrome. This includes a combination of NSAIDs, jaw joint physiotherapy exercises and bite raising appliances (often described by patients as "mouth guards" Fig 6.2) to try to relieve jaw joint pressure points. Increasingly, specialist care is arranged in an MDT format. Referral should be either to the patient's dentist, or a routine referral to OMFS. It is important to remember that surgery is only rarely indicated so conservative treatment is often the mainstay and can easily be delivered in a primary care setting in conjunction with local dental input.

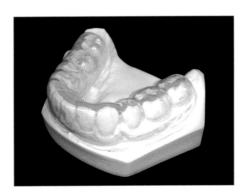

*Fig 6.2: A soft lower bite raising appliance used to treat TMD. Image courtesy of Mr Lawrence Dovgalski and the Maxillofacial laboratory, Morriston Hospital, Swansea, UK.*

FACIAL PAIN / ALTERED SENSATION

## TRIGEMINAL NEURALGIA

The symptoms of trigeminal neuralgia are well described. Classically it produces a sharp 'lightning' like pain in the distribution of one or all of the divisions of the trigeminal nerve (ophthalmic, maxillary, mandibular, Fig 6.3) and typically occurs in 'bursts' lasting seconds at a time, though the pain can last for hours or even days at a time. The pain often has a specific trigger, i.e. touch or temperature, and does not cross the midline. On examination there is usually no sensory loss to the associated nerves. Referral to OMFS is warranted to rule out an organic cause for the pain, and an MRI is performed to assess for the presence of a space-occupying lesions compressing the trigeminal nerve root ganglion or any evidence of multiple sclerosis. Once the above are excluded, it can be managed successfully in primary care with analgesia and anticonvulsants, such as carbamazepine, which have been shown to be effective. Cryotherapy or nerve decompression can be considered for refractory cases.

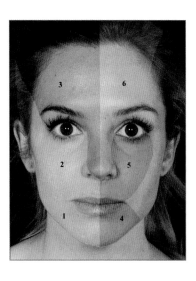

*Fig 6.3: Trigeminal nerve sensory innervation of the face (right side) and regions supplied by terminal sensory nerves that are potentially amenable to interventional procedures by the maxillofacial surgeon (left side).*

1. *Mandibular division of the Trigeminal nerve (V3)*
2. *Maxillary division of the Trigeminal nerve (V2)*
3. *Ophthalmic division of the Trigeminal nerve (V1)*
4. *Mental nerve*
5. *Infraorbital nerve*
6. *Supraorbital nerve (and supratrochlear nerve)*

## ATYPICAL FACIAL PAIN AND BURNING MOUTH SYNDROME

In contrast to trigeminal neuralgia, atypical facial pain and burning mouth syndrome represent facial pain syndromes with no organic cause and a strong psychological component.

The pain and symptoms of atypical facial pain follow no myofascial or nerve distribution, varying in character and with no recognizable pattern, and crucially do not disturb eating or sleep. Commonly, patients with atypical facial pain have a preceding psychiatric history but it should be appreciated that this is not always the case. As a diagnosis of exclusion, routine referral to OMFS will serve to rule out an organic cause, and antidepressants can be tried and monitored in primary care.

In a similar fashion burning mouth syndrome produces pain affecting the oral cavity, with altered taste (often metallic) and the perception of a dry mouth (subjective xerostomia) but no identifiable cause. Before specialist referral to OMFS, blood tests should be ideally sent to assess

FACIAL PAIN / ALTERED SENSATION

for haematological and nutritional deficiencies including FBC, B12, folate and ferritin. Infective causes, such as candidiasis, can also lead to oral discomfort. Tricyclic antidepressants have been shown to be effective in these patients.

## REFERRAL TO DENTIST

### DENTAL PAIN

As discussed, dental pathology is still the most common cause of facial pain.

As decay on the tooth surface begins to spread into the tooth the symptoms may be of a sharp/sensitive pain that lasts for seconds and may not be easily localised to the offending tooth. If this progression continues and the decay reaches the nerve (pulp) within the tooth, then the pain turns into a dull ache that lasts minutes to hours and is more localised to the tooth. This is the sequence of 'pulpitis'. Once the infection spreads from the pulp down the roots of the tooth to the bone, there is a constant pain, with a tooth that is tender to touch and biting (this is termed 'periapical periodontitis', Fig 4.12). From here the infection will suppurate, either draining to the gum surface as a gum boil (see Chapter 4), or forming a fascial space collection with ensuing facial swelling and systemic upset. From the above it can be seen that dental pain normally progresses in a stepwise fashion and with a good history you should be able to differentiate this from other causes of orofacial pain.

It may seem obvious that a patient with dental pain will attend a dentist and not their general medical practitioner. However, the time course between pulpitis and a facial swelling may be protracted, and for those patients who have poor oral hygiene or a dental phobia, dental pain is a common occurrence often ignored. It may be only the presence of significant pain or sepsis that will prompt their attendance.

FACIAL PAIN /
ALTERED SENSATION

## IMMEDIATE REFERRAL TO ON-CALL OMFS

In a systemically well patient, with no signs of facial swelling then referral to the patient's dentist is of course appropriate. Any signs of sepsis, significant swelling, acutely intolerable pain, restricted mouth opening and/or concern over the airway should prompt an immediate referral to the local on-call OMF surgeon. *See Chapter 4 for more information on spreading orofacial sepsis.*

## OTHER CAUSES OF FACIAL PAIN AND ALTERED SENSATION

You should always have in the back of your mind the differential diagnoses of facial pain that require referral to other specialties; for example a space-occupying lesion, temporal arteritis or multiple sclerosis. These presentations and appropriate referral pathways should be well known to every Primary Care Clinician.

FACIAL PAIN / ALTERED SENSATION

# CHAPTER 7: RESTRICTED JAW MOVEMENT

## INTRODUCTION

The temporomandibular joint is a complex region of the facial skeleton. It is comprised of the condylar head of the mandible, the glenoid fossa at the base of skull, a cartilaginous disc separating an upper and lower compartment, each filled with synovial fluid, surrounded by an overlying joint capsule (Fig 7.1). Furthermore, joint pain and the ability to open and close one's jaw is also reliant on facial musculature and other related soft tissues. Whilst most problems opening and closing the jaw will be related to benign pathology related to the joint or surrounding musculature, occasionally restriction in jaw movements can alert the clinician to more sinister causes.

### ASK:
- Onset of symptoms: gradual vs sudden?
- Getting worse?
- Pain – diffuse (e.g. muscular in temporalis/masseter) vs localized (e.g. TMJ), associated with jaw clicking/crepitus/movements
- Risk factor assessment
- Previous trauma to jaw/known facial fracture?
- History of tooth grinding (bruxism) or parafunctional habits (e.g. chewing gum)
- Stress or other psychological problem?
- Does the patient feel that there has been a change in their dental occlusion

## LOOK:

- Can they fully open their mouth, what is the maximal inter-incisal opening?
- Can they fully close their mouth, does their bite feel normal for them?
- Palpate muscles of mastication – masseter, temporalis, lateral & medial ptyergoids
- Palpate for lymphadenopathy
- Intraoral examination – signs of bruxism (e.g. tooth wear, scalloped tongue, frictional keratosis on cheeks), swellings/ ulceration (malignancy), abnormal consistency of soft tissues (submucous fibrosis).

## SINISTER FEATURES:

- Abnormal intraoral findings (e.g. swelling/ulceration)
- Lymphadenopathy
- Nerve involvement (altered sensation or weakness), otalgia
- Progressive/ rapidly worsening symptoms or trismus
- Risk factor history (smoking, alcohol, betel nut chewing)

RESTRICTED JAW MOVEMENT

# DO: MANAGEMENT ALGORITHM

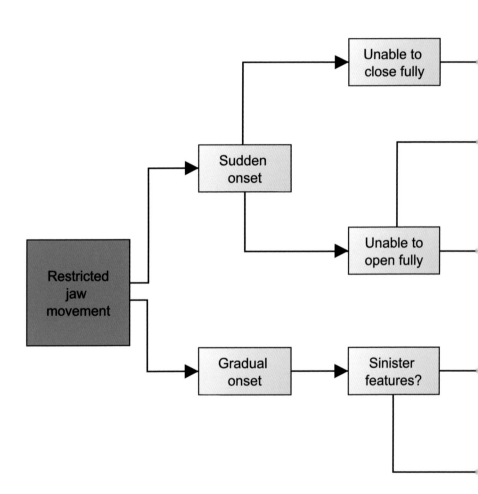

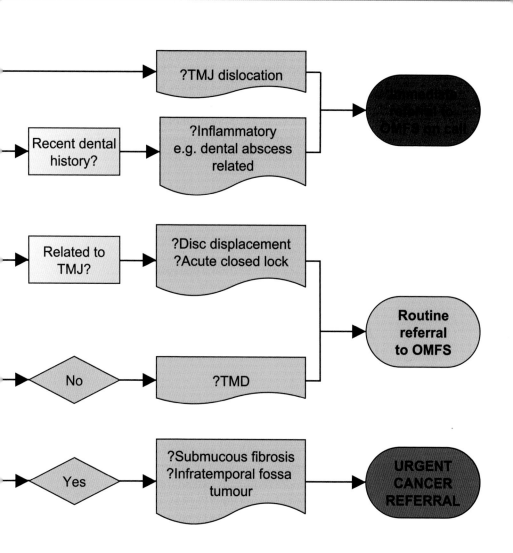

## URGENT CANCER REFERRAL

Patients with submucous fibrosis can develop progressive significant restriction in their mouth opening. These patients often have a history of chewing betel nut, which is often carried in the buccal pouch, leading to a chronic inflammatory response and progressive fibrosis in the submucosal and deeper connective tissue layers. These lesions, which result in stiff oral mucosa with visible white fibrous bands giving a marbled appearance (Fig 3.4), are premalignant and as such require prompt referral for assessment. In rare cases, severe disease may require management for nutritional support due to oral dysfunction. *See Chapter 3 for more information.*

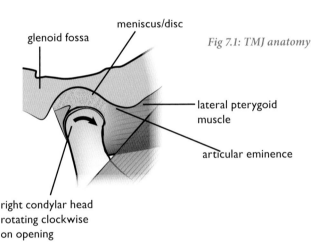

glenoid fossa

meniscus/disc

*Fig 7.1: TMJ anatomy*

lateral pterygoid muscle

articular eminence

right condylar head rotating clockwise on opening

Tumours in the infra-temporal fossa region can also lead to restriction in jaw movement by interfering with the joint itself or the muscles responsible for jaw movements. Tumours can either arise primary in the infra-temporal space or more commonly extend from adjacent areas such as the nasopharynx or maxillary antrum (Fig 7.2). This anatomical region is difficult to access and is closely related to vital structures including the orbit, cavernous sinus and internal carotid artery, making management difficult. However, from the primary care perspective, the key is to recognise any associated sinister features enabling the Primary Care Clinician to choose between an urgent cancer referral versus a routine referral pathway.

RESTRICTED JAW MOVEMENT

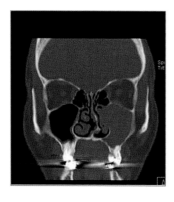
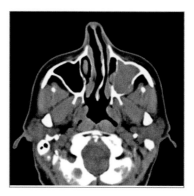

*Fig 7.2: A tumour of the left maxillary antrum, beginning to erode through the posterior antral wall and into the infratemporal fossa with potential future involvement of masticator muscles.*

## ROUTINE REFERRAL TO OMFS

Once a suspicious diagnosis has been excluded, difficulties in jaw, opening both of gradual and sudden onset, can most likely be attributed to temporomandibular joint dysfunction (see TMD page 67), which in itself is a complex range of presentations. A brief overview of the mechanism of jaw opening can help with understanding these presentations at primary care (Fig 7.3)

A sudden change in a patient's ability to fully open their jaw, often associated with a history of an audible click can suggest disc displacement. However, the history and extent of the opening deficit can be extremely varied (Fig 7.4).

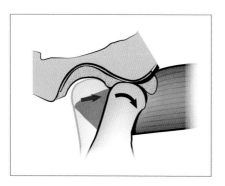

*Fig 7.3: Diagram of normal jaw joint movement in relation to condylar head and disc. As well as rotation (black arrow) on mouth opening the condylar head slides forwards on the meniscus/disc (red arrow)*

RESTRICTED JAW MOVEMENT

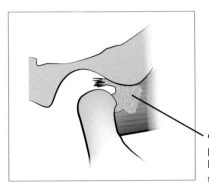

*Fig 7.4: Diagram demonstrating abnormal anterior displacement of the disc, restricting translation of condylar head and therefore mouth opening.*

disc detached
posteriorly and
bulging anterior to
the condylar head

Gradually progressive symptoms are difficult to assess, particularly as TMJ dysfunction can be related to numerous, and often overlapping, factors - distorted joint anatomy or mechanism of jaw movement, effect of surrounding musculature and parafunctional habits (e.g. tooth grinding, chewing gum) as well as psychological influences. A thorough history and examination can help elucidate the causes of the disease and the direction of onward referral. Treatment options for the vast majority of patients will be conservative and include maintenance of a soft diet to limit workload on the jaw, jaw exercises and the use of soft bite guards by the local dentist to control the effects of bruxism on the jaw joint. It may be prudent to try these management techniques prior to referral to secondary care, where further imaging techniques such as dynamic (mouth opening and closing) TMJ MRI will provide more detailed information about the joint anatomy. Further management is only warranted in selected cases but would include botulinum toxin injection into masticatory musculature, TMJ arthrocentesis and arthroscopy along with open joint surgery.

RESTRICTED JAW
MOVEMENT

# IMMEDIATE REFERRAL TO ON-CALL OMFS

Patients who present with a sudden onset inability to close their jaw with their mouth in a wide-open position will most likely be suffering with a dislocated TMJ, where the condylar head has slipped forward over the articular eminence (Fig 7.5). Patients are often distressed and report previous similar episodes. The earlier the jaw is relocated, generally the easier the procedure is to carry out. While unusual to present in primary care (these patients often make their way straight to the emergency department), providing the history and examination findings are consistent with simple spontaneous dislocation (with no acute history of trauma which may have caused a fracture-dislocation of the condyle) there is little harm, provided the clinician has appropriate experience, in attempting to relocate the jaw in the practice setting. If unsuccessful they can be sent to the local OMFS on-call team. Otherwise, the patient should attend the emergency department as soon as possible as an increased duration of dislocation will make simple closed reduction of the joint more difficult due to masticatory muscle spasm (and they may require intravenous sedation or even GA with muscle relaxant to achieve joint reduction).

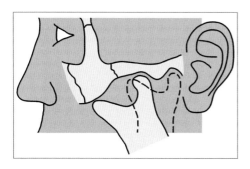

*Fig 7.5: Anatomical representation of the dislocated condyle leaving the glenoid fossa to lie anterior to the articular eminence*

RESTRICTED JAW MOVEMENT

# CHAPTER 8:
# NECK LUMPS

## INTRODUCTION

A patient presenting with a neck lump is not uncommon. Most of the diagnoses and referral pathways discussed below will be familiar. However, what may be unfamiliar is the requirement to look in the mouth should a possibly sinister neck lump be found.

**ASK:**

- Duration (< / > 3 weeks?)
- Getting larger?
- Painful?
- Aesthetic concerns?
- Associated symptoms e.g. mouth ulcer etc.?
- History of infection/discharge?
- History of foreign travel?
- Cat scratch recently (toxoplasma)?
- 'B symptoms?' (fever, night sweats, unexplained loss of weight)?
- If in region of major salivary gland – mealtime symptoms?

## LOOK:

- Site and size – where is it in the neck? If midline, does it move on swallowing/tongue protrusion?
- Single or more than one
- Shape, surface and edge – smooth or irregular?
- Colour
- Consistency – Soft v hard (possible metastatic disease) or rubbery (lymphoma)
- Fluctuance
- Attached to skin/deep tissue?
- Signs of infection?
- Palpate the rest of the neck for cervical lymphadenopathy (check other nodal sites also)
- Examine the mouth and oro-pharynx.

## SINISTER FEATURES:

- Fixity to underlying structures
- Hard or rubbery consistency
- Multiple firm nodes
- Rapidly enlarging
- Hoarse voice / dysphagia
- Irregular edge
- Nerve involvement (altered sensation or weakness)
- Rapidly increasing in size
- Strong risk factor history
- Oral/oropharyngeal swellings/symptoms

NECK LUMPS

# DO: MANAGEMENT ALGORITHM

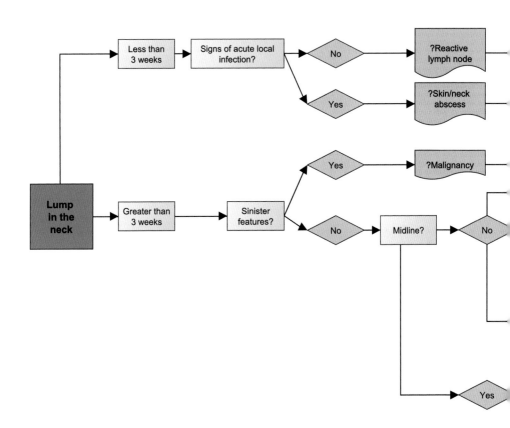

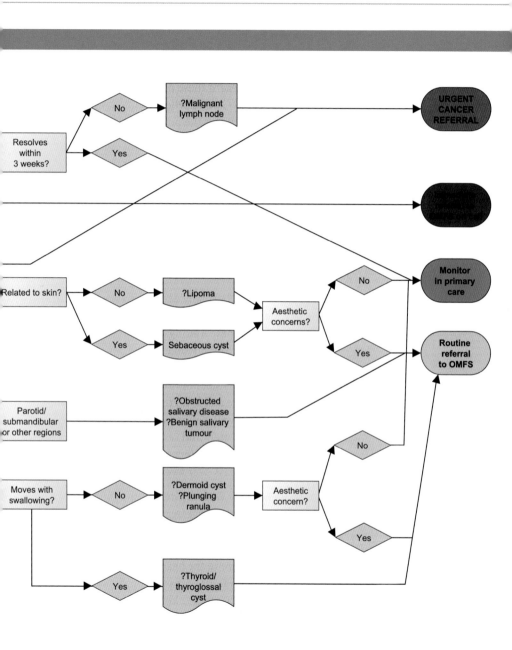

Broadly speaking, the assessment of a neck lump is based on the consideration of a number of factors, namely: site, tissue origin, chronicity and risk factors. The above flow diagram attempts to provide a framework to guide your thought process with regard these diagnostic factors. As per UK National Institute for Health and Care Excellence Guidelines, our flow diagram starts with a cut-off of 3 weeks for the presence of a neck lump. The management/referral decision is based upon the location and the presence of any sinister features.

# URGENT CANCER REFERRAL

## CERVICAL LYMPHADENOPATHY

For the purposes of this book, the goal is the recognition and safe referral of suspected cancer.

A palpable malignant lymph node is classically described as being hard or rubbery, progressing to a matted fixed mass with an irregular edge, and being larger than 1cm (Fig 8.1). These findings relate to the irregular growth of the cancer within the node and possible spread beyond its capsule in to the adjacent tissue (Fig 8.2). In contrast a reactive lymph node (lymphadenopathy secondary to infection/inflammation) exhibits hyperplasia of normal lymphoid tissue and is therefore contained within its capsule and presents as a firm but well-defined and mobile mass. The reactive lymph node should appear acutely and resolve as the infection subsides i.e. within 3 weeks, whereas the malignant lymph node will present as a progressively enlarging mass over weeks to months.

The combination of lymphadenopathy with sinister features and strong risk factors should prompt an urgent cancer referral to the one-stop neck lump clinic, which in most units is run jointly with ENT and OMFS. It is important to remember that over 90% of metastatic cervical lymph nodes will have a primary tumour somewhere in the head and neck, so a general enquiry of head and neck cancer symptoms and a thorough examination of the oral cavity is mandatory (see Chapter 1). You should be aware of the basics of lymph node levels of the neck (page 7), which will aid the accuracy of your referral and may focus your examination: for example a submental/submandibular (level I) lymph node will commonly point to an ipsilateral

NECK LUMPS

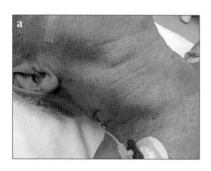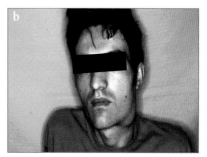

*Fig 8.1 (a) Metastatic SCC causing right level I and II palpable lymphadenopathy.*

*Fig 8.1 (b) Tuberculous cervical lymphadenopathy*

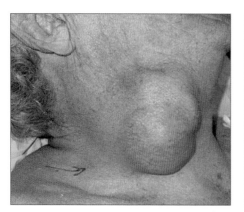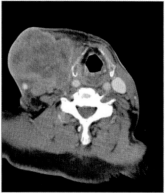

*Fig 8.2: Large neck metastasis from tongue cancer after failed radiotherapy*

mouth cancer, and the presence of spread to contralateral or higher level lymph nodes carries a poorer prognosis.

Other causes of lymphadenopathy should also be considered. A reactive lymph node can resolve as a fibrotic node that remains chronically enlarged. Lymphadenopathy in a child, or with the presence of 'B' symptoms (fever, night sweats, unexplained weight loss) or itching in an adult should raise concern; referral in this case will be governed by the patient's history.

NECK LUMPS

Finally, you have an important role to play in the follow-up and surveillance of head and neck cancer patients. Whilst patients with locally advanced tumours commonly have an elective neck dissection, the management of stage I disease (N0-node negative) is controversial. Therefore, the surgeon may opt for primary resection (with/without extensive lymph node resection) and surveillance through serial follow-up appointments. Seeing the patient on a regular basis, perhaps for other diseases, you might be the first to palpate a malignant lymph node in between their routine follow up appointments and save valuable time.

## IMMEDIATE REFERRAL TO ON-CALL OMFS

The urgency of referral of a neck/cervical skin lump, will be governed by the presence of infection (See Chapter 4; neck space infections, Fig 4.11). A suspected neck space abscess should be discussed immediately with the local on-call OMF surgeon. Signs such as decreased mouth opening, change in voice, drooling and inability to swallow should raise concerns over an impending airway compromise and in this case an emergency call for an ambulance is appropriate. Smaller, localised skin abscesses, such as an infected 'sebaceous' (epidermoid) cyst, can be discussed with the on-call surgeon and may be amenable to review on a dedicated clinic for review and possible incision and drainage.

## ROUTINE REFERRALS

### SKIN LUMP

The management of a sebaceous cyst, lipoma or other benign skin lesion will be determined based largely upon aesthetic concerns, and the patient can be informed of this, perhaps negating the need for referral (Fig 8.3). The referral of skin cancers is covered in Chapter 5.

NECK LUMPS

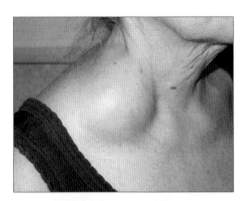

*Fig 8.3 a) Lipoma of the neck*

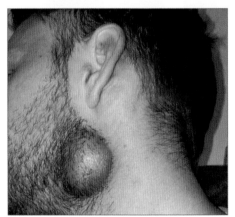

*Fig 8.3 b) An infected epidermoid ("sebaceous") cyst of the neck*

## SALIVARY, THYROID AND OTHER NECK MASSES

These presentations will not discussed in detail. Within this category the location of the lump will often be the main diagnostic factor. Patients with a clear history of salivary obstruction and/or sialadenitis (in the absence of sinister features) can be referred routinely.  Acute salivary infection can be treated accordingly with antibiotics.

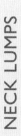

NECK LUMPS

However, a tail of parotid mass can be difficult to distinguish from a neck lesion and should always be treated suspiciously (Fig 8.4). Unless there is a clear benign history, an urgent cancer referral is indicated, even though the majority will turn out to be benign tumours (remember that the larger the salivary gland, the smaller the chance of malignancy). Although uncommon, parotid swellings with facial nerve palsy or any other sinister features are of course of grave concern and warrant urgent cancer referral (Fig 8.5).

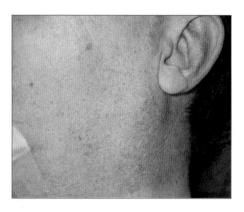

*Fig 8.4: A subtle swelling of the parotid tail which turned out to be a Warthin's tumour. Such lesions can be smooth and difficult to discern from level II neck nodes on clinical examination alone.*

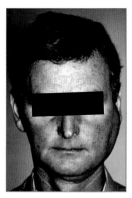

*Fig 8.5: A malignant parotid tumour with a clinically-subtle weakness of the buccal branch of the facial nerve (loss of the left nasolabial fold and depression of the left upper lip).*

## MONITOR IN PRIMARY CARE

If the diagnosis of a neck lump is obvious and benign, such as a resolving reactive lymph node or a simple skin lesion, then reassurance and monitoring in primary care is safe and appropriate. A routine referral can be made at a later date should the patient wish to discuss further treatment.

NECK LUMPS

# GLOSSARY

Ameloblastic carcinoma – a histologically malignant epithelial tumour arising from dental enamel tissue.

Ameloblastoma – a benign tumour of dental enamel tissue which can exhibit moderately aggressive growth.

Aphthous ulcer (simple) – a simple oral ulcer, painful and present for distinct duration (less than 3 weeks).

Bruxism – the 'parafunctional' habit of subconscious tooth grinding, thought to be associated with stress and often thought to commonly occur at night.

Dentigerous cyst – an odontogenic cyst arising from the embryological follicle of an unerupted tooth. Classically the cyst lining arises from the neck of the tooth at the cemento-enamel junction. This cyst grows and commonly expands cortical bone and displaces adjacent teeth.

Dentoalveolar – pertaining to tooth-bearing 'alveolar' bone.

MDT – multidisciplinary team.

Malignant ameloblastoma – histologically an ameloblastoma but exhibiting very aggressive growth (including soft tissue seeding and/or locoregional metastasis).

Masseteric hypertrophy – enlargement of the masseter muscles. Often idiopathic in nature but in some cases associated with bruxism/stress.

Myofascial – pertaining to muscle and fascia (as a source of jaw joint pain for example).

Odontogenic keratocyst – an odontogenic cyst containing keratin. This cyst is less inclined to displace teeth and expand the jaw (although it may) but rather silently tends to spread along the medullary cavity of the jaw and can therefore be extremely large at presentation.

Parafunctional habits – non-physiological habits of jaw joint movement (e.g. excessive chewing of gum, bruxism, posturing of the mandible into non-resting positions.

Periapical cyst – a cyst originating from a chronic periapical abscess/periapical granuloma (secondary to dental sepsis). This is classically sited over the apex of the causative root. It often expands cortical bone and displaces adjacent teeth.

Recurrent aphthous stomatitis (RAS) – an autoimmune condition of repeated ulceration of the oral mucosa. Lesions eventually disappear completely but recur in a similar form later.

# INDEX